COULD YOU BE SUFFERING FROM ANXIETY DISORDER AND NOT EVEN KNOW IT?

Anxiety affects millions of people, and the signs can be more subtle than you think. You don't have to be someone who trembles at the thought of social interaction or is unable to keep a job because of obsessive hand washing or counting aloud.

The following patients were recently diagnosed with an anxiety disorder:

- Jill, age thirty, a costar in a television sitcom who lives in fear that her mind will go blank and she will forget her lines
- Sam, age forty-one, a well-known criminal-defense attorney who suffers from sleep disorder and fear of flying
- Matt, age twenty-seven, a bright doctoral student with a family history of phobias who has a fear of heights and social interaction.

This is the new face of anxiety disorders. If you see yourself reflected in these descriptions, know that there is hope. Like these patients, you can achieve a happy, stable life naturally—without drugs—if you begin to learn . . .

WHAT YOUR DOCTOR MAY NOT TELL YOU ABOUT ANXIETY, PHOBIAS, AND PANIC ATTACKS

WHAT YOUR DOCTOR MAY *NOT* TELL YOU ABOUT™

ANXIETY, PHOBIAS,

AND

PANIC ATTACKS

The All-Natural Program
That Can Help You Conquer Your Fears

DOUGLAS HUNT, M.D.

WARNER BOOKS

NEW YORK   BOSTON

The title of the series What Your Doctor May *Not* Tell You About . . . and the related trade dress are trademarks owned by Warner Books and may not be used without permission.

Warner Books

Time Warner Book Group
1271 Avenue of the Americas, New York, NY 10020

Visit our Web site at www.twbookmark.com.

Printed in the United States of America

First Edition: November 2005
10   9   8   7   6   5   4   3   2   1

Library of Congress Cataloging-in-Publication Data
Hunt, Douglas
      What your doctor may not tell you about anxiety, phobias, and panic attacks : the all-natural program that can help you conquer your fears / Douglas Hunt.— 1st ed.
         p. cm.
      Includes index.
      ISBN 0-446-69181-X
   1. Panic disorders—Popular works. 2. Phobias—Popular works. 3. Anxiety—Popular works. 4. Self-help techniques. I. Title.
   RC535.H863 2005
   616.85'22—dc22

                                                        2005005032

This book is dedicated to Jeanne Manning for her tireless efforts in tediously reading and rereading the manuscript for corrections. Her "schoolteacher" comments made my job harder but more rewarding. The book is also dedicated to Debra Fulghum Bruce, Ph.D., who spent an inordinate amount of time reviewing and polishing the material. I also want to dedicate this book to my wife, Mary Hunt, who allowed me the time it takes for research, as well as writing. And, finally, thank you, Denise Marcil, my literary agent, for bringing this opportunity to me. Thanks, to all four of you wonderful ladies.

Contents

Preface

⎯⎯⎯⎯⎯⎯⎯⎯⎯

This is a book about fear—and how to control it naturally. Fear is a tremendous handicap. Although it may not be a physical one, obvious to all, it is a disability and it affects millions. Fear is an intense sense of "substantial uncertainty" and it manifests itself in many ways with anxiety, stress, phobia, panic, nervousness, hypervigilance (acute awareness of your surroundings), and excessive worry.

The tragic events of September 11, 2001, reminded all Americans of our vulnerability, both as a nation and as individuals. Yet beyond the nagging fear of terrorism, each day we are confronted with more stressors—whether from job loss, divorce, death of a loved one, a rebellious teenager, caring for an elderly parent, or being diagnosed with a chronic illness. We all feel fear more now than ever before—and we are overwhelmed. Overpowering fear can incapacitate you just as much as blindness or a broken leg. Not only does fear disable motivation, it inhibits our ability to think clearly, make commitments, solve problems, and act decisively. Fear robs us of doing our best work and affects our quality of life; we can't experience any of life's pleasurable feelings when our stomach is in knots. Pervasive and intense uncertainty interferes with strong relationships, job performance, and social life. Fear is a challenging disability.

You might wonder why I make so much of redefining fear or describing uncertainty as a disability. That's because most people don't appreciate the damaging effects created by chronic fears such as developed anxiety disorders, panic, sleep problems, and more, and won't (or don't) take the appropriate actions to control these fears. I've seen people suffer with anxiety and worry for years before they finally give in and admit that something has to be done; fear is ruining their life.

For many of us, the only step we take to overcome fear is to see a doctor or therapist and get a prescription for some kind of medication and not much else—not even an explanation of how the drug works or its possible side effects. However, I know that drugs are *not* the long-term solution to the problem of fear. You don't have to take pills to recover from anxiety and panic disorders. I've learned this from more than thirty years as a practicing psychiatrist, treating anxiety, fears, phobias, and panic attacks without drugs.

Granted, some of us are born anxious; and others become anxious as a result of situational stress or threat to one's life, property, or relationships. The good news is that anxiety is a potent motivating force for needed change and a vital quality for survival. Yet, like all forces, anxiety can get out of hand and begin to do more harm than good. At that point, at the point of excess, we describe anxiety as a disabling disease.

Billions of dollars have been spent searching for a solution to disabling anxiety. What causes this disease is much simpler to answer than what perpetuates it. There is no doubt that fear causes physical changes, permanently or semipermanently. The drugs related to anxiety all reflect the changing viewpoints of scientists regarding what really perpetuates it. For example, the psychiatric view of the cause for chronic anxiety is multifaceted, including:

- genetic factors
- neurotransmitter excess or deficiency
- memory disturbances
- anatomical organ deficits in critical areas of the brain
- adrenergic over-activity

Yes, this list is long and grows daily, as does the conveyer belt of new drug applications seeking approval because of the inadequacies of our current medications. While each new drug approaches the problem of anxiety from a different perspective, most pharmaceuticals that resolve anxiety come with a lengthy list of side effects.

Perhaps that's one reason a growing number of Americans are exploring alternative or natural therapies for relief of mild anxiety and associated problems, even as the potential benefits of conventional pharmaceuticals seem to improve. Seeking a healing relationship between patient and health care provider, these men and women hold true to the philosophy that natural or less invasive therapies can optimize a person's innate healing capacity. The best health care is based in good science, and it is also open to new paradigms and promotes the appropriate use of more natural, less invasive treatments whenever possible.

In 2003 alone, more Americans visited an alternative therapist (about 600 million) than a primary care physician and spent their own money for this opportunity (about $30 billion). Annually, we spend about $250 million a year on homeopathic remedies, and more than $4 billion on natural dietary supplements, including herbs. Yet how is a person to know which of these alternative treatments are safe and effective? And what about conventional medications? Can prescribed pharmaceuticals even with all their rigorous testing be trusted to promote healing without causing undesirable side effects? (After all, more than 100,000 deaths a year occur in U.S. hospitals because of adverse reactions to common medications.)

There are credible answers, and this book provides them.

I wrote this book to present a *revolutionary program* for ending anxiety disorders and living fear-free with natural therapies that are substantiated by modern science without being inhibited by it. For this very reason, my 5-step program is multifaceted and focuses on many natural therapies and lifestyle changes rather than one answer to relieve anxiety disorders. I believe in addressing the mind, body, and spirit in a way that is effective, reasonably priced, and free of adverse side effects.

With formal training as a psychiatrist, I practiced as one for years before I transitioned from a drug-dominated conventional approach into a natural, complementary one. For more than thirty years, I have been practicing alternative and preventive integrative medicine. Integrative medicine is a method of healing that focuses on health rather than on disease, the oneness of mind and body, and the ability of the body to heal itself with the proper support. To do this, I utilize a considerable variety of nonprescription agents to improve health problems, including those involving mental health. I believe that the doctor and patient should work in partnership, employing therapies that support the natural capacity for healing we all possess.

The key to this book may be found in these few words: *Mental stability reflects physical stability*: *un*reasonable anxiety is a form of mental instability, often stemming from impaired physical health. Physical health is not exclusively organ health; it includes biochemical efficiency, and physiological and even genetic function. This book will help you to search out physical weaknesses and eliminate them. Sleep, energy, hormone balance, and immune strength, among others, all influence physical health and, ultimately, mental stability. Drugs can control anxiety, but so can a stronger and healthier body!

In this book, I provide you with my 5-step holistic program filled with practical and action-oriented alternative solutions and information for recovery. You are about to learn some simple lessons and explore some tools that will free you from your burden. Fear is an emotional disability, but I know it is one you can overcome.

Finally, this book is not meant to take the place of one-on-one therapy. Read it, take copious notes, and then make an appointment with your doctor to talk about the natural solutions that might help your situation. Good luck!

Douglas Hunt, M.D.

WHAT YOUR DOCTOR MAY *NOT* TELL YOU ABOUT™

ANXIETY, PHOBIAS,

AND

PANIC ATTACKS

Part 1

UNDERSTANDING ANXIETY

Chapter 1

What Your Doctor May *Not* Be Telling You

Picture someone who suffers with an anxiety disorder. Do you immediately think of a withdrawn recluse who trembles at the thought of social interaction? Perhaps you envision a neurotic young man who cannot hold a job because of obsessive-compulsive behavior such as constant hand washing or counting aloud.

I want you to imagine the following patients who were recently diagnosed with an anxiety disorder in my clinic:

- Jill, age thirty, a rising young actress and costar in a television sitcom who lives in fear that her mind will go blank and she will forget her lines.
- Sam, age forty-one, a well-known criminal attorney who suffers with sleep disorder and fear of flying.
- Carmen, age fifty, a boutique owner and mother of four whose husband ran off with a young business colleague without any warning, leaving her with feelings of rejection and fears of abandonment.

- Matt, age twenty-seven, a bright doctoral student with a family history of anxiety and phobias who has a fear of heights and social interaction.

The truth is that most people wouldn't associate these men and women with having an anxiety disorder. But these people reflect the new face of anxiety disorders. Perhaps you even see yourself in their descriptions.

I've successfully treated these adults—and thousands more—from a host of anxiety disorders that used to engulf them in fear, phobias, panic, and obsessions. Today, they live happy, stable lives and have learned natural ways to alleviate the anxiety and cope with the uncomfortable symptoms.

OUR ANXIOUS NATION

If you or a loved one suffers with an anxiety disorder, you are not alone. The latest surveys show that more than 20 million Americans suffer from an anxiety disorder in any given year and another 30 million will have the problem at least once during their lifetime. From panic, fears, and phobias to obsessive-compulsive disorder and post-traumatic stress, anxiety manifests in mysterious ways and does not discriminate by age, gender, or race. Statistics indicate that specific phobias lead the list with 6.3 million people affected, and panic disorder affects another 2.4 million.

No matter what type of anxiety disorder you or a loved one might have, you know it can plague all aspects of life: your marital and family relationships, productivity and ability to earn a good living, sleep, eating habits, exercise and activity, and overall well-being.

While anxiety disorders impose a high personal burden,

they are costly to society as well. Anxiety sufferers utilize up to a third of every dollar spent on health care in the United States, with doctor visits at nearly $22 billion a year. Along with emergency care, prescription drugs, and hospitalization, we have lost productivity, absenteeism, and a combination of malingering and genuine discomfort.

Anxiety disorders don't just disappear overnight. They usually are chronic problems and are just as disabling as any physical ailment. In the most severe cases, depression and suicide attempts often follow long-term unresolved anxiety.

Besides living with the burden of a chronic, dysfunctional state, the anxiety patient often endures a lack of respect for having this disease. Many physicians reflect societal prejudice that anxiety patients simply suffer from a flawed character. Despite the prevalence of significant psychiatric disorders, fewer than one in three adults ever seek help for this problem. And, when they do seek help, it's often for another medical reason and therefore confusing to the health care provider.

Very often, the first time a doctor sees a patient suffering from anxiety, the presenting symptom is a physical complaint. For instance, post-traumatic stress disorder (PTSD) patients often seek help for cardiovascular, neurological, respiratory, or musculoskeletal problems. During a doctor's consultation, they rarely mention anxiety unless the physician discovers the underlying problem and mentions it first. Generalized anxiety disorder (GAD) patients often seek help for nonspecific pains in the chest, which they believe to be angina or heart-related. Many anxiety patients see themselves as being less physically and psychologically capable than others and may even perceive themselves as having a disability.

UNDERSTANDING ANXIETY DISORDERS

The word "anxiety" means to anticipate future danger or misfortune, internal or external, and to be apprehensive about it. The body reacts to these thoughts by creating physical tension and significant discomfort. Throughout this book, I'll be talking about anxiety at a level exceeding that of the average person's distress, to a point where anxiety has become a disease. There are certain criteria that must be met if a condition is to be designated an anxiety disorder:

1. There must be significant mental distress; and
2. There must be impairment in the social, work, or other important areas of daily life.

When we categorize anxiety, this does not mean that nothing else may be going on. Categorizing by similarities is one method of organizing and nothing more. All of those patients who constitute a category are still people with different personalities and possibly other emotional or physical problems. The classifications of these disorders are strictly for clinical, educational, and research purposes. In reality, it has become part of a system necessary for third-party payment and various legalities. Perhaps, more than anything else, the system provides a method of communication between participants in the health system.

The official *Diagnostic and Statistical Manual of Mental Disorders* is commonly used as a guideline for diagnosis of anxiety, phobias, panic, and stress-related problems. However, as a physician, I believe that this manual is not the be-all and end-all when it comes to making an accurate finding. If you expect absolute precision in the diagnosis of an anxiety disorder, you will be disappointed, as there are no specific boundaries to encompass this type of disorder. That's because there are so many perspectives from which to view anxiety, including distress, adaptability, self-control, disability, inflexibility, irrationality, cause, a measure of deviation, and so on. There also is a great deal of leeway in the present diagnostic system, allowing room for a clinician's personal opinion. The openness of the system does not leave gaps as one might think, but rather it allows for greater flexibility. In other words, the experienced clinician can exercise her own personal judgment as to what she is seeing and treating with the patient.

To summarize, nothing is black-and-white in the present system of diagnosis for anxiety disorders. Many patients come to see me because they have already seen three to five health care professionals and are discouraged by a lack of concrete diagnosis or by what they suspect to be a misdiagnosis of their anxiety problem. They are also frustrated by the resultant ineffective treatment. With most medical problems, we are used to a laboratory test that determines the exact problem and medication that treats that problem. But there is no specific laboratory test or exact medication that will end anxiety disorders quickly. Rather, it takes time for you to work with your doctor to narrow down the diagnosis and then use trial and error to find the exact pharmaceuticals or nutrients that work with your body's chemistry to resolve the problem. I always remind patients that the boundaries of each type of anxiety disorder are flexible. This fluidity is primarily due to the many theories as to how people become ill. I will cover this more throughout the book.

ANXIETY KNOWS NO BARRIERS

As stated, anxiety knows no barrier in age or gender. In addition, increasingly more children today harbor high anxiety, which can lead to depression or other disabilities. The onset of anxiety at a young age, combined with some depression and moodiness, can significantly affect schoolwork and sabotage academic success. For instance, in findings published in August 2003 in the journal *Archives of General Psychiatry*, researchers set out to determine the level of disability in children incurred by problems such as anxiety. A representative sample of participants was followed for six years to measure the disability that occurred secondary to psychological symptoms. The authors identified three areas that were specifically affected, including family, school, and peer relationships. They concluded that boys had more trouble in school, while girls had more problems with their family. The childhood anxiety was as likely to result in disability, as was depression.

In a follow-up study, 1,420 children ages nine to thirteen were assessed annually for a psychiatric disorder until they were sixteen. During that period, 13.3 percent of the participants had at least one psychiatric disorder (panic, depression, anxiety, social anxiety, or substance abuse), although it was not necessarily chronic or long lasting. Girls, in particular, seemed to cycle back and forth from anxiety to depression. The authors concluded that the risk of a child having at least one psychiatric disorder by age sixteen is much higher than previously suggested and that girls are more likely to be affected.

Although the initial cause of anxiety may emanate as much from family situations as from other factors, the existence of the anxiety state further destabilizes all other aspects of a youngster's life. If the trigger that initiates the anxiety is particularly severe stress, then the victim may feel as if her life has changed forever.

Older Adults

Anxiety rears its ugly head among older adults as well, with 15 percent of older men and women reporting anxiety symptoms (feeling fearful, tense, or nervous). Moreover, 43 percent of those with depression experience anxiety, according to research published in the April 2003 issue of the *Journal of the American Geriatrics Society*. In this particular study, 3,041 patients were asked if they experienced at least two episodes a week of intense anxiety. The results were no surprise—they did. Other studies have indicated a higher incidence of anxiety. If there were difficulties with hearing, or if they experienced incontinence, hypertension, or poor sleep (common in the elderly), the number of patients reporting anxiety increased significantly. Patients whose social functioning was poor and who needed extra emotional support were more likely to have greater and often chronic anxiety symptoms.

It is believed that anxiety in the elderly may be a better predictor than depression of eventual dementia. One illuminating study published in the July 2002 issue of the journal *Medicine and Science in Sports and Exercise* revealed that chronic anxiety might lead to memory impairment, further cognitive decline, and finally senility.

Lifetime Relevance

Although intense anxiety is commonplace in modern-day urban life, it is not considered a disorder until it interferes with normal activities. If you don't have an anxiety disorder, you might wonder what your risk is of developing one in the future. Here are some of the latest statistics:

- 25 percent chance of an anxiety disorder
- 2 to 3 percent chance of a panic disorder
- 4 to 5 percent chance of agoraphobia
- 3 percent chance of obsessive-compulsive disorder
- 13 percent chance of social phobia
- 11 percent chance of any specific phobias
- 7 to 8 percent chance of post-traumatic stress disorder

MY PROBLEMS WITH DRUG THERAPY

So, if you are diagnosed with an anxiety disorder, you simply pop a pill to alleviate it, right? Wrong! While some anxiety disorders respond to pharmaceuticals, there are short- and long-term adverse effects to be considered that can often be more crippling than the disorder itself. In addition, pharmaceuticals are extremely costly compared to natural therapies, which are usually found over-the-counter at your local health food store. My holistic program will show you a safer, cheaper, and more effective way to strengthen the body and increase wellness, and in doing so, reduce anxiety.

When I started my practice in the 1960s, pharmaceuticals were usually reserved for hospitalized patients and psychotics. Of course, there were many other modalities available then, and I'll get to them in a moment. But first I want to share with you my initial experiences with psychotropic drugs, which explain why I resisted the pressure of joining other doctors in embracing prescription drugs as mainstream psychiatric therapy.

Keep in mind that "psychotropic" and "psychoactive" have

virtually the same meaning and are often interchangeable words. They describe a drug, generally used to treat mental illness, which has the ability to alter moods, anxiety, behavior, thinking processes or mental tension.

Short-Term Side Effects

I'm a prime example of someone whose body and mind are not the least bit compatible with mind-altering drugs. For example, if I take a stimulant such as a mild appetite suppressor or even a cup of coffee, I will develop tachycardia (rapid heartbeat) and an arrhythmia (irregular heartbeat) that lasts anywhere from hours to days. This is dangerous, to say the least—not to mention unpleasant. When I am in this altered, medicated state, I am unable to focus my thoughts or do any constructive work. If I ingest a tranquilizer (a downer), I am zonked out for a day and a half.

To give you an idea, when I was an intern, I once took a 10 milligram (mg) Valium (diazepam), a commonly prescribed class of drug called benzodiazepine, before going to work. After taking this anti-anxiety agent, I literally was unable to get off the couch for a full day. I had to call in sick—the only day of my entire internship that I missed. Psychoactive drugs and I simply do not get along.

Many of my patients have experienced the same adverse effect with benzodiazepines. Along with the drowsiness, they have reported slurred speech and dizziness. One patient, thirty-two-year-old Victoria, said she was unable to wake up until noon after taking medication the night before for mild anxiety. When she awoke, she discovered that her two preschoolers had unlocked the front door and were playing in the front yard near a busy highway. I'm sure Victoria's mild anxiety turned into outright panic when she thought of what could have happened to her unsupervised young children.

Another woman, Caroline, age forty-seven, took Valium to help ease anxiety during a lengthy divorce. She came to me for a natural therapy, saying the tranquilizer made her so numb that she was devoid of all emotions. "The drug calmed my anxiety," Caroline said, "but after taking it for a week, it also dulled any joy or enthusiasm I had for life."

People who do not have problems with drugs are often puzzled by or suspicious of those who say they can't take mind-altering medications. To them I say, why not see this for what it is—one extreme along the spectrum of responses to chemicals. At the other extreme are those who never feel normal without drugs. These people can easily become abusers. In between, we find the average person, who can tolerate the majority of drugs pretty well. Still, there is more to the problem of taking drugs than simple tolerance.

Long-Term Adverse Effects

Along with the short-term uncomfortable side effects of drug therapy, there can be long-term adverse effects that can sometimes be toxic. Any drug that acts on the central nervous system (such as an analgesic, a stimulant, or a depressant) is potentially able to cause noxious side effects such as cognitive impairment, dependence, habituation, or neurological disorders. In fact, up to 10 percent of patients using psychotropic drugs report serious side effects, including hepatitis, dermatitis, low white blood cell count, amnesia, paradoxical excitation, changes in vision, hearing alterations, breathing problems, hypertension, low blood pressure, fast or slow heartbeat, palpitations, and headaches, among others.

Today there are thousands of studies on the toxic effects and resulting adverse reactions to psychotropic medications. There are hundreds of studies on suicides, overdoses, and deaths from use of these drugs, not including driving accidents and memory impairment.

Drug therapy for anxiety usually consists of using anti-panic drugs for immediate symptom relief while attempting to find the most appropriate mix of drugs from several different categories, including antidepressants, anti-seizure and anti-anxiety medications. Yet, drugs, and especially psychotropic drugs, are not as specific in their actions as you may think. For example, the benzodiazepines (tranquilizers such as Valium, Ativan, and Xanax) have five major therapeutic qualities:

1. Anxiety reduction (anxiolytic)
2. Hypnotic (sleep-inducing)
3. Muscle relaxant
4. Anti-epileptic
5. Amnesic (ability to ignore or forget unfavorable events)

Benzodiazepines such as Valium act by enhancing the effects of gamma-aminobutyric acid (GABA) in the brain. GABA is a neurotransmitter, a chemical that nerves in the brain use to send messages to one another. GABA inhibits activity in many of the nerves of the brain, and it is thought that this excessive activity is what causes anxiety or other psychological disorders. Patients who take this class of drug may be subject to all of the above-mentioned treatment actions, along with any other adverse effects that may result, including rebound anxiety or insomnia (a major surge of anxiety or insomnia immediately after a drug that controlled the anxiety or insomnia is discontinued), aches and pains, epileptic seizures, and memory problems, among many others. In fact, most people are unaware that more than 500 different types of adverse reactions to benzodiazepines have been reported to the FDA. Because there are so many chemical effects and because benzodiazepines are fat-soluble and thus remain in the body, no part of the body or brain is exempt. Yes, the expected benefit may occur with these medications; but there is always the potential for an enhancement of any preexisting psychological or physical problem in addition to possible new problems.

Virtually every doctor recognizes individual variability in therapeutic and adverse effects. For example, a strong prescription might affect you and yet have no effect at all on a family member. Benzodiazepines accumulate in the body and brain at different speeds and different levels in each person.

With the long-term use of psychotropic drugs, mental and emotional impairment, if it occurs, comes on gradually and is often barely noticed by the patient. It is of interest to note that patients who have become dependent on the drugs are unlikely to ever respond normally to those drugs again, once they are discontinued.

Big Pharma Promotes Expensive Options

Prescription drugs are driven by what is known as Big Pharma, the big-business pharmaceutical industry. In fact, many of the so-called latest and greatest breakthrough medical studies are funded by the pharmaceutical industry and thus the outcomes reported can sometimes be biased. Deserved or not, Big Pharma often gains power and respectability from the government through lobbying and financial contributions. Consequently, legislation and government agencies such as the Food and Drug Administration often reflect the interests of these companies.

Most doctors get their drug information from well-paid sales reps who work for Big Pharma and don't have time to explore other remedies, specifically the healing benefits of natural (and inexpensive) therapies that are less known. These doctors have little time to explain the possible risks of these medications to patients or to teach them key lifestyle changes that might benefit the patient's overall health.

This is problematic because the consumer often receives pricey and sometimes ineffective pharmaceuticals when a natural therapy might work just as well and cost a lot less without all the deleterious side effects. Natural approaches often do not make big money for powerful drug companies and do not get the testing, FDA approval, and the million-dollar advertising budget that drugs produced by Big Pharma receive.

Post-Withdrawal Symptoms After Long-Term Benzodiazepine Use

During the 1980s, there were substantial long-term studies related to latent physical and psychological symptoms (see pages 13–14) that resulted from discontinuation of psychotropic drugs. The effects were not exclusive to acute withdrawal but also were seen after discontinuation of long-term benzodiazepine use.

These symptoms would not be occurring had there not been a semipermanent or even permanent change in the brain's neurochemical or neurological system. While it is true that some people who use psychotropic drugs do not

experience post-withdrawal symptoms, the risk is still there
for many others.

- behavioral disorders
- bursting head feeling
- delusions
- depression
- gastrointestinal problems
- headache
- increased anxiety
- insomnia
- irritability
- malaise
- moodiness
- neck tension
- neuromuscular problems
- numbness in extremities
- palpitations
- panic
- paranoia
- perceptual difficulties
- phobias
- poor concentration
- sensory disturbances
- shaking and trembling

THE MENTAL HEALTH SYSTEM BEFORE DRUG THERAPY

The mental health system did not always rely on pharmaceuticals for treatment. During my residency, psychiatric treat-

ment was focused on helping patients gain insight into their problems. It was believed that insight would eventually translate into behavioral changes favorable to a happier and more productive life.

I did my residency on a farm. I'm not kidding! The California mental health system was originally created around the concept of a self-sufficient facility, and it worked beautifully. The idea was for patients to play a large part in their own recovery. Patton, Napa, Camarillo, Norwalk, and other mental hospitals were actually self-sufficient farms.

During the daytime hours, patients were assigned work. During off-work hours, they could be active in the many recreational facilities. Patients worked in every department of the facility, tending farm animals, working in the fields, or performing maintenance work, depending on their individual abilities.

In the evening hours, patients enjoyed movies or activities such as baseball, tennis, horseshoes, basketball, or dozens of other games around the grounds. Traditionally, patients were required to attend group therapy or, when there was sufficient staff, other forms of therapy during the week.

Patients spent their days engaged in productive but simple activities. At the end of the day, they had something to show for their efforts; they had created an orderly and hygienic environment. Besides keeping their minds off their problems, the tasks they performed encouraged a real sense of self-enablement. Moreover, there was also a huge cost savings here for the mental health system. Because the patients were contributing to their own upkeep, the burden on taxpayers was reduced.

Today, the California mental health system's approach differs vastly from its former communal treatment methods. And, in my opinion, the current therapies that favor medications and behavioral modification often leave patients less able to function in society than before. For example, those patients who are the most mentally handicapped often become homeless. They become easy prey to drug dealers and other bottom-dwellers who also inhabit this dangerous environment.

I was fortunate to have participated in a successful but long-forgotten system of mental health that did not rely entirely on drugs. So, when I began my private practice in the 1960s, I gravitated toward more natural approaches. Early in my practice, I found an article on nondrug approaches to mental health written by Dr. William Philpot, a psychiatrist then practicing near Boston, Massachusetts. Dr. Philpot was kind enough to invite me to spend time with him so I could observe his nondrug modalities. I also drove to Connecticut to see Dr. Marshall Mandell, a psychiatrist, now retired. Dr. Mandell introduced me to the idea that food sensitivities could influence mental stability. I met with Dr. Theron Randolph, another expert, who practiced in Chicago, Illinois. Dr. Randolph graciously allowed me to watch him interview patients for environmental influences on their mental status.

In observing these gifted physicians, who favored natural therapies over prescription drugs, two things struck me immediately: One, the natural approaches they used were successful in helping patients. And, two, each one spent a great deal of time with each patient. Dr. Randolph, for example, spent as many as four hours performing a single intake interview. Instead of looking at each patient's obvious symptoms, the doctors would search for the patient's uncommon, individual characteristics and then connect them to a possible causative agent or situation. Taking such care and time in reviewing patients' unique situations became a cornerstone of my methods.

Still not convinced that natural was necessarily better or

safer, I continued to dabble in these alternative therapies on patients with milder cases of anxiety. Some patients took the natural treatments along with a reduced dose of medication and were pleased with the relief they felt. Others were able to give up pharmaceuticals altogether as the natural modalities eased their anxiety and gave them a better quality of life. I also experimented with a host of alternative and lifestyle modalities such as diet, exercise, hypnosis, biofeedback, and magnets. Gradually I began to coalesce the many ideas that I had collected along with my own ideas into a solid plan to benefit my patients—especially anxiety patients. Moreover, for the most part, my plan avoided the use (and misuse) of conventional drugs.

Almost all of my patients on the natural therapy plan responded in a positive way and were pleased that these inexpensive alternative therapies were effective but with fewer side effects. As these patients shared success stories with family and friends, more and more people heard of my holistic treatment plan, and my practice started to expand, which is why I'm writing this book today.

MY 5-STEP HOLISTIC PROGRAM

Since my first experiences, learning from brilliant doctors and holistic therapists who used natural modalities for psychiatric illnesses, I have gained invaluable insight in how to treat anxiety disorders without potentially dangerous pharmaceuticals. I wrote this book to put *you* at center stage by focusing on the many alternative modalities that I've found to work.

The 5-step holistic program in this book is neither intrusive nor does it include mind-altering drugs that reduce energy and productivity. As you read the book, you'll see that it quickly moves beyond the descriptions of common types of anxiety disorders on to pages of natural, self-help tips that you can use today to feel more relaxed, worry less, and be more productive. This multifaceted program is the same one I recommend to patients and will give you the most effective low-tech, natural approaches to stopping mild anxiety and reversing related disorders without deleterious side effects.

In the thirty-five years that I've been in practice, we've had many successes. Working closely with my patients, we've learned what works and what doesn't. I share all of this information with you in the pages of this book, including how making a few small changes in lifestyle habits can give tremendous anxiety-relieving results.

In the upcoming chapters, I will discuss the various types of anxiety disorders as found in the official *Diagnostic and Statistical Manual of Mental Disorders*. As you read this first section of my book, I will help you identify the particular type of disorder you might have, understand the risk factors and symptoms, and then discuss the diagnosis and treatment in the holistic program to follow. It is important to note, however, that while the various expressions of anxiety may differ, the core problem is always the same. In some cases, dealing directly with the primary symptom is the key to recovery. But, in many, if not most, of the other forms of anxiety, simply addressing the anxiety itself is sufficient for reducing the symptoms and returning to full health.

I believe that this book is the next best thing to consulting with you in person. Therefore, in preparation for the 5-step program, I want you to take the test "Assess Your Risk for Anxiety Disorders" and evaluate your own risk factors. If you already have an anxiety disorder that is stealing your productive life, this test will help you see what you need to do to recover as fully as possible and to prevent the disorder from recurring.

ASSESS YOUR RISK FOR ANXIETY DISORDERS

Take a few minutes to identify your personal risks and symptoms for anxiety disorders. The following questions are similar to the ones I ask patients who come to my office for a consultation. Give yourself one point for each time you respond with "yes." Add up your score at the end of the questionnaire and use the key to interpret your score.

1. Do you suffer with anxiety around the clock, during all waking hours?
2. Are you easily "set off," irritated, or frightened?
3. Do you harbor sensitive feelings, and see everything as a perceived threat?
4. Does anxiety make your inner life hell?
5. Has anxiety influenced your daily life to the extent that you sleep poorly, over- or under-eat, have urinary frequency, or smoke too much?
6. Has anxiety taken all of your energy so that you feel chronically tired?
7. Are you so desperate for relief that you have turned to alcohol?
8. Has your anxiety caused those around you to respond with anger, irritability, impatience, or avoidance and even rejection?
9. Has your intellectual performance declined because of poor memory, concentration, or task stamina?

10. Has your career or job performance fallen significantly because of your anxiety?

11. Are you suffering much more than anyone around you suspects?

12. Is your mind racing from one worry to another and thus complicating most of your everyday obligations?

INTERPRETING YOUR SCORE:

1. **0: Superb!** You have no signs or symptoms of anxiety disorders. Following the lifestyle suggestions in this book should help you stay healthy.

2. **1–3: Low risk.** You have a low risk of anxiety disorders. Still, review the areas where you responded with a "yes" and modify your lifestyle accordingly.

3. **4–6: Moderate risk.** You have a moderate risk of anxiety disorders. My program will enable you to get back in control of negative lifestyle habits and decrease the chance that anxiety disorders will overwhelm your active life.

4. **7–12: High risk.** Though you might not feel as if anxiety has taken over your normal life, you are at a high risk for having problems with this illness. Read this book and learn all about the various anxiety disorders. Also, evaluate your personal lifestyle to see what habits need to be changed. Consider the natural therapies as you strive toward a healthy mental state.

NOW, LET'S GET STARTED!

As you read this book, you'll meet many of my patients who have successfully conquered some debilitating anxiety disorders with my holistic program. Just like them, your goal is to change the habits you can control so that you greatly reduce the chance of having anxiety overwhelm you.

Throughout these pages, I will help you get focused so that when you talk to your doctor, you can explain clearly what you are experiencing with anxiety. However, before I discuss the many natural therapies and lifestyle habits for relieving anxiety, let's look at signs and symptoms you might feel, as discussed in Chapters 2 and 3. I want to help you get back in control of your active life without the burden of anxiety—and understanding the problem is the first step.

———— ❧ ————

Chapter 2

Anxiety, Phobias, and Panic Disorder

If you suffer with symptoms of anxiety, phobias, or panic disorder, you are not to blame—and you are not alone. Especially in our modern society, which grows more complicated and frustrating every day, anxiety disorders are commonplace. In fact, 6 percent of men and 13 percent of women in the United States have an anxiety disorder, according to a recent survey by the National Institutes of Health Epidemiologic Catchment Area, and medications are standard treatment. Many of my own friends and colleagues rely on one or more medications so they can ease anxiety and function productively.

I myself use the nutritional supplements I prescribe for my patients. For instance, I use my stress spray during daytime hours to stay relaxed and fall asleep easily at night. I believe that most people would choose a natural remedy over a medication, if only they knew about the options. The problem is, most people don't know exactly what's out there or how to distinguish between and take advantage of the many supplements lining natural food store shelves. Here's where my book comes in.

ANXIETY IS COMMONPLACE

One patient of mine—we'll call her Judith—said her anxiety began around the time of the terrorist attacks on September 11, 2001. Although this young magazine editor was shy most of her life, Judith suddenly became fearful of every new situation. Instead of going to clubs or shopping with friends on weekends, Judith had extra deadbolt locks put on her door and spent long hours in her small Manhattan apartment, peering out the window for anything suspicious. When asked to travel abroad with close friends, something Judith normally enjoyed doing, she quickly made up an excuse to avoid being put in a precarious situation of another possible attack.

Finally, it came to the point where Judith could not walk down the streets of Manhattan to her daily editing job without experiencing rapid heart rate, breathlessness, and a sense of numbness or disorientation. She took a leave from her job and lived with a close friend until she regained her confidence again.

When a person suffers anxiety, fear colors everything around them. The greater the level of anxiety, the greater the fear of common hazards—hazards that seldom bother others. You don't have to live this way! Treatment for anxiety disorders is readily available. Still, many people like Judith avoid seeing a doctor or they fail to disclose their problems to the doctor honestly—and completely miss an active life.

After the terrorist attacks on September 11, a survey of physicians showed a significant increase in prescriptions of anti-stress medications. During this same time, doctors referred vastly more patients out to counselors than in previous years. Today, the number of people who are actively being treated for anxiety is just the tip of the iceberg. Yet countless people with similar levels of anxiety are suffering silently like Judith, afraid that their symptoms might be dismissed as trivial, afraid that they will be blamed for their problem altogether.

Anxious adults are not the only victims. Kids are fast approaching adult numbers when we consider the frequency with which they are placed on drugs. According to data published in the January 2003 issue of the journal *Archives of Pediatrics and Adolescent Medicine*, children are two to three times more likely to be given psychotropic medication now than they were in 1987, and these numbers are escalating.

Another comprehensive study of 3,242 youths between the ages of fifteen and nineteen, reported at the 2003 American Academy of Child and Adolescent Psychiatry, reveals that 36 percent of the participants reported a lifetime history of at least one period of depression for at least two weeks. Many of the adolescents told of having years of depression. Anxiety and related problems know no barriers in age or gender.

As we grow up, there are the normal states of anxiety that are universal. Preschoolers find certain objects or situations frightening. In grade school, fears focus more on physical harm and health. Adolescents agonize over social adequacy and performance. Within this enormous pool of kids growing up are some who are more sensitive than others. In fact, some experts believe that 10 to 15 percent of all children are anxious enough to be classified as having an anxiety disorder.

In addition to the group that falls within the normal range, you might question if there's a more extreme group outside the spectrum. Can it be that genetically predisposed individuals, who are more vulnerable, become more anxious than others under approximately the same levels of stress? I'll try to answer this question as I further explain the specific disorders.

UNDERSTANDING ANXIETY DISORDERS

Anxiety disorders are the most common psychiatric disorders. Because no one can predict the future, some level of worry is normal and will always exist. Yet, undeniably, certain events suggest a greater chance of loss than others. Personal security, important relationships, freedom, or rare opportunities all may be uncertain and become a cause of great concern. The level of value you place on the unsettled circumstance or event determines your level of anxiety. While everyone worries about uncertainty, at least one out of seven people suffer from chronic anxiety.

In this book, I discuss a variety of anxiety disorders, which include phobias, fears, panic attacks, and stress-related maladies, among others. But first, let's look at the difference between the terms "anxiety," "fear," and "stress":

- *Fear*—a distressing emotion aroused by impending danger.
- *Anxiety*—a distressed mind caused by the fear of something.
- *Stress*—an emotional tension caused by something frightening that may also destabilize the physiology of the body.

The term "stress" includes the element of physiological change. However, other than that difference, fear, anxiety, and stress are very similar in meaning, and all three are frequently interchanged in scientific literature.

In my mind, the terms "fear" and "anxiety" are the same, and any attempt to separate their meaning would be splitting hairs. The word "stress" may be used in place of "anxiety" with complete accuracy, but it may also be used when describing a stress-induced ulcer because of prolonged anxiety. The term "stress" is a broader term because it has been used in scientific fields other than psychology or medicine. For example, engineers use the term "stress" to describe metal fatigue, meaning a weakening of the metal parts of machines.

Different Definitions for the Same Problem

Anxiety, pure and simple, is a normal reaction to stress. A little anxiety is motivating. It helps you perform well at work or on an exam and to work harder to achieve your goals. However, when anxiety gets away from itself, it begins to take on a life of its own. While anxiety may be generated initially from legitimate stress or fears, it can transform itself into a perpetual loop where there are never any moments of peace. Once you reach this point, your molehills become mountains, and the anxiety is out of control.

When anxiety skyrockets, you must work to solve two problems:

1. You must eliminate the initial problem (the stressor or trigger); and
2. You must eliminate your newly acquired fear-machine whose cycles now dominate the nervous system.

A precise definition of anxiety has yet to be determined. That's because so many physical phenomena have been discovered that a consensus is currently impossible. For example, suppose a group of blind people were trying to describe an elephant, having only examined one small part of it. Naturally, each of them would offer a different description. Likewise, scientists define anxiety according to the results of their own particular studies. The problem is that they have all been studying different aspects of the same disease.

As we discuss the different types of anxiety disorders in this book, you will gradually see how blurry the borders become. For example, fear of flying appears to be a simple phobia on the surface and would seem to call for a specific remedy. However, the person with a fear of flying is often an overly vigilant person who worries excessively about many other things. The core problem in all of these disorders is an unhealthy amount of anxiety.

I believe that it's the underlying anxiety that drives its form of expression—whether with panic disorder, fears, or phobias. Yet, the form of disorder that emerges from the basic anxiety depends entirely on the person. The form of anxiety, be it a phobia or social withdrawal, depends mostly on a person's adaptive mechanism plus their genetic proclivities. It's common for the anxious person to drift between categories of anxiety, or even straddle one or more.

What Causes Anxiety?

Anxiety has various causes about which scientists have hypothesized extensively. One group of experts says that anxiety is caused by disruptions in the normal balance of brain neurotransmitters, involving a failure of proper cellular communications.

Others in the scientific community emphasize the size and activity of specific areas of the brain that relate to the different anxiety disorders. Whether it is the limbic system, the group of brain structures that are involved in emotions such as aggression, fear, and pleasure and in the formation of memory, or the hypothalamus, which regulates hunger, thirst, and sexual re-sponse, the dysfunctional area clearly is associated with the state of anxiety. Any increase in activity in the locus ceruleus, the nucleus in the brain stem responsible for the physiological reactions involved in stress and panic, will cause anxiety. Like-wise, a decrease in activity in the locus ceruleus decreases anx-iety.

Another group of scientists believes that the different branches of the sympathetic nervous system or the part of the autonomic nervous system that accelerates the heart rate, con-stricts blood vessels, and raises blood pressure, and the chemi-cals most closely associated with that system, are the culprits of anxiety.

I could go on with more theories and textbook jargon, but I am sure you get the picture. Just like the blind people trying to describe the elephant without seeing it, each of these de-scriptions represents one piece of the puzzle of what the beast looks like.

Who's at Risk?

Anxiety is thought to stem from a complex mixture of genetic, environmental, psychological, and bodily factors. While anxi-ety is its own event, it may be greatly influenced by related in-ternal functions such as lack of energy, hormone instability, and poor diet or health, to name a few. Fluctuations in these and other natural functions act as triggers to anxiety or inten-sify existing anxiety. It makes sense that if these stated condi-tions can influence anxiety negatively, then by manipulating the same or similar features properly, we can influence anxiety in a constructive way and, hopefully, reduce it.

Since anxiety can be chemically induced in a nonanxious

individual, it is clearly possible for a physical problem to produce anxiety without a psychological component. For instance, an overactive thyroid (hyperthyroid) can easily produce the physical state of anxiety regardless of the person's mental state. Poor sleep can cause the symptoms of anxiety as well.

Whether you are genetically at risk for high anxiety or whether you acquired it over time, it's important to deal with anxiety before it gets out of control. Harboring high levels of anxiety for extended periods often deteriorates into something more serious like depression.

Signs and Symptoms

Your body's early warning system promotes anxiety as an "alert" so you can actively counteract and successfully manage the problem at hand. However, *anxiety itself* is a negative and painful feeling. With anxiety, you might have one or more of the following physical symptoms:

- racing or pounding heart
- excessive worry and over-diligence
- easy sweating
- trembling or shaking
- shortness of breath
- feeling of being smothered
- chest pains
- knots in the stomach
- unsteady or light-headed sensations
- numbness or tingling

When anxiety gets high, it can undermine sleep, energy, and other physical strengths and can paralyze productive activity. Anxiety worsens other mental problems such as depression. High anxiety can seriously color judgment and may cause inappropriate actions that worsen the problem.

To say that someone has significant anxiety is tantamount to saying the person has a disability; *they are one and the same.* The only question is whether the disability is mild, moderate, or severe.

There are many forms of anxiety, including phobias and panic disorder. The medical and psychological professions have classified various forms of anxiety with the expectation that each type, once recognized, will lead to treatments for that form of the disorder. However, specific antidotes for each are less focused than psychiatrists and psychologists would like you to believe. While classification is useful for communication and documentation, for the most part, physicians simply write prescriptions for anti-anxiety medications for any and all forms, based upon whatever they've found useful in their own experience.

Let's look at the major types of anxiety. Later in the book, I will describe the various diagnostic and treatment protocols that I use in my clinic.

GENERALIZED ANXIETY DISORDER (GAD)

Generalized anxiety disorder (GAD) is excessive worry that permeates all areas of life and is characterized by a minimum of six months of persistent anxiety. With GAD, the intensity, duration, and frequency of the worries are *significantly out of proportion* to the actual likelihood of damage from a feared event.

When anxiety becomes a handicap, it has crossed the line from normal to abnormal. For example, GAD reaches that point when the *anxiety itself* begins to preoccupy your thoughts and darkly color most of your decision-making. At that point, anxiety can:

- Reach the level of a disability.
- Distract or even paralyze your thoughts and actions.
- Place stress on your metabolism.
- Alter normal physiology to the extent that it may graduate into diseases such as ulcers or hypertension.
- Affect the central nervous system and the sympathetic nervous system.
- Affect muscles throughout the body.

Perhaps the most striking characteristic of GAD is how easy it is to become fearful yet how difficult it is to overcome.

Who's at Risk?

There are literally hundreds of ways one can become anxious and fearful, and you already know most of them. In the case of GAD, there is a 20 percent risk among blood relatives of people with the disorder and a 10 percent risk in those with clinically depressed relatives. A sleep disorder may cause anxiety just as anxiety may lead to sleep problems.

Those with a family history of GAD are also susceptible. An interesting study on twins was published in the July 2003 issue of the journal *Archives of General Psychiatry*. In this study, researchers measured the twins' fear responses by electrodermal skin conductance, a biofeedback measure that gives feedback of changes in skin conductance. The authors found that with the models in this experiment, there were two sets of genes that influenced the tendency to be fearful. One gene relates to the process of the habituation of the fear and the second gene connects to the process of associating the fear with an object or situation. Researchers concluded that a third to half of the subjects' fear-conditioning process could be ascribed to genetic influences rather than environmental factors.

Signs and Symptoms

With GAD, you might be overly concerned about work, finances, relationships, family, health, past failures and future concerns, and the fact that you have no control over the constant anxiety. In addition to the worries, people with GAD have trouble sleeping and are irritable and tired most of the time.

Most patients suffering from GAD find that excessive worry occurs more days than not. As for the present, they worry about the fact that they have no control over their pervasive anxiety. For a proper diagnosis of GAD, you must have at least three of the following signs and symptoms:

- muscle tension
- fatigue
- restlessness
- poor concentration
- irritability
- difficulty sleeping

Patients who suffer from GAD experience worries that are out of proportion to the reality of a given situation. It's relatively common to find this type of patient also suffering from bipolar disorder (also called manic-depressive disorder). Bipolar disorder is a medical condition that causes extreme mood changes that alternate between episodes of depression and mania or elation. GAD patients sometimes show symptoms of hypochondria, in which they focus on imagined physical ailments, with complaints such as dry mouth, nausea, lump in the throat, diarrhea, urinary frequency, difficulty swallowing, nervousness, stuffy nose, and more.

Diagnosing Generalized Anxiety Disorder

Review the following questions to see if you are at risk of GAD:

1. Are you constantly worried or overly concerned about matters both large and small?
2. Do you find it difficult to stop worrying?
3. Are you frequently restless or on edge?
4. Is it often difficult to concentrate?
5. Do you suffer broken sleep?
6. Are you both tired and irritable at the same time?
7. Are you seriously concerned you may have a hidden disease?
8. Would you or someone who knows you say you are a nervous person?

If you answered yes to any of these questions, talk to your doctor about your anxiety concern and seek an accurate diagnosis. There are many natural therapies and lifestyle habits discussed in my holistic program that may help you. Discuss these with your doctor to see which ones work best for your situation.

Anxiety or Agitation?

Agitation or a high level of uncontrolled excitement within the body and mind often ends up in aggression and that can quickly reach the level of a psychiatric emergency. In the worst cases, doctors are forced to administer several drugs together such as Risperdal (risperidone) and Ativan (lorazepam) to rapidly dissipate the explosive energy. In thirty or forty minutes, most patients come under control again.

Agitation is more recognized in the acute stages and less so when it is mild to moderate. At the lesser levels it may be confused with more recognized forms of anxiety or may even be present at the same time there is another form of anxiety present. When agitation plays a role in the discomfort, the usual anti-anxiety nutrient will not be very effective, as the muscles are more involved. However, both magnesium and antioxidants (pages 137–138 and 139–144) can be effective in targeting and relaxing muscle tension due to agitation.

PHOBIAS

Phobias are common anxiety problems and strike one out of ten Americans, with women twice as likely to have a phobia as men. Phobic individuals have an unreasonable or irrational fear of something that poses little or no real danger, whether a situation, object, or event. Understandably, they avoid this perceived danger as much as they can. Nevertheless, if they can't avoid what they fear, then it immediately provokes a marked anxiety response such as rapid heartbeat, nausea, or profuse sweating.

Such responses can even escalate to the point of a panic attack (see pages 45–48). People of all ages can suffer panic attacks, but while children do not immediately recognize that a fear is exaggerated and generally unreasonable, adolescents and adults do.

The phobic patient may have a seemingly reasonable cause for his unreasonable fear (such as having been bitten by a dog or surviving a plane crash). The problem is that the person's level of fear is highly exaggerated. With a phobic fear, the anxiety is worsened by the thought that you might lose control if faced with the dreaded situation. This worry greatly accentuates the fear.

Another related component of a phobia is the question of distance from the feared object or situation. A dog at a distance may not elicit much fear, but the closer the patient comes to the dog the more fear escalates. In many cases, simple phobias are not disabilities, since the feared object is rarely encountered. For example, a city-dweller who is phobic about snakes may never even see the dreaded reptile. The phobia becomes a moot point. On the other hand, a salesman with a fear of flying or a postman phobic about dogs might find that their phobia interferes with job performance.

There are five subtypes of phobias:

1. Animal
2. Environmental (lightning, storms)
3. Blood, from an injection and/or an injury
4. Situational
5. Other rare types such as fear of wealth, ugliness, or snow

In many cases, a person may have multiple phobias of different subtypes, although most of the time the phobia is from the same subtype group.

Cultural fears (magic, spirits) are not considered to be a phobia unless they significantly alter that individual's lifestyle as mentioned above. Children frequently go through a transitory stage of semi-phobias, but this is not abnormal unless it persists. Alternatively, if the child reaches a point where, for example, he cannot be coaxed to school for fear of meeting a dog on the way, the fear is considered irrational.

Who's at Risk?

Phobias often begin in childhood and continue into adult life. If this is the pattern, only about 20 percent of patients will experience a spontaneous remission. Most of the time phobias must be actively treated if they are to be overcome. There is a mild connection to genetic influences because immediate family members tend to suffer from the same phobia subtypes.

Some phobias stem from a traumatic incident. Yet they may also stem from repeated warnings from parents about a specific object or situation. For instance, thirty-year-old Rob remembers his mother warning him about lightning and thunderstorms to the point that he gave up being on the neighborhood sports teams for fear a sudden storm would approach. While a healthy fear of lightning is normal, to this day, Rob has a phobic fear of lightning and avoids outdoor activities during summer months with family and friends.

Signs and Symptoms

When it comes to phobias, overlapping symptoms frustrate a clear-cut diagnosis. It is not uncommon to end up with a mixed diagnosis such as agoraphobia, social phobia, and specific or animal phobia.

The number of people in this country who have phobias ranges from 6 percent up to as high as 20 percent, depending upon which reports you read. Most serious phobias are often considered a component of another more severe mental disturbance such as a bipolar disorder. Regardless of the prevalence of your particular phobia, if you have one, the discomfort is difficult to bear.

In my practice, I rarely see a patient just for a simple or specific phobia like fear of dogs or snakes. When such fear emerges, it's almost always during an exam for a much broader level of anxiety. I do see many cases of fear of heights and social phobia. Still, the most common phobia I have found is fear of flying, and even then, it is usually in conjunction with another form of anxiety. If patients want to completely neutralize a simple phobia, they must be desensitized, and I'll discuss how to do that using nutrients later in the book.

Fear of heights is different from fear of flying. While most people don't fly that often, they do find themselves in high places almost daily, whether buildings, bridges, ladders, or hillsides. The next most common phobia that I see is social phobia.

SOCIAL PHOBIA

The key element to social phobia is the marked and persistent fear of social or performance situations, especially if there is a possibility of embarrassment. The fear that precedes the situation is one level of anxiety (anticipatory anxiety), but the second level appears when the victim is exposed to that situation. At this time, the fear may move up to a full panic attack with symptoms like fear of losing control or fear of dying.

Most people who live with a social phobia recognize that it

is an unreasonable fear, but they simply can't control it. Part of their fear stems from the worry that others will judge them or dislike them. Additionally, they often fear that others will see their shaking hands and hear their unstable voice and know they are afraid. An important distinction is that phobias differ from paranoid delusion, which is when one holds a false belief despite evidence to the contrary. Examples would include delusions of grandeur or persecution, or a somatic type such as hypochondriasis, a somatoform disorder characterized by severe anxiety over having a disease.

Being fearful before public scrutiny does not warrant the diagnosis of social phobia. A little stage fright is normal, and may even provide a useful edge. In contrast, a person who is socially phobic is unable to engage in normal social activities without experiencing almost a panic level of fear. Such fears may occur in almost all social situations, or they may be narrowed down to only a few. In the case of generalized social phobia, one has to question the patient's social skills and whether this may be a form of agoraphobia, a fear of being in places or situations that are potentially embarrassing.

If a diagnosis is in doubt, there is one laboratory test that can be performed to distinguish social phobia from panic disorder. Social phobics do not, as a rule, experience panic attacks if given sodium lactate IV or carbon dioxide by inhalation as do panic patients. Talk to your doctor to see if this test is used in your area.

Most social phobics have a variable level of fears, depending on the circumstance. This hierarchy of fear levels reflects the average person's reaction to different conditions. For example, like many people, social phobics may have a greater level of fear when speaking publicly than while socializing in a small group.

Risk Factors of Social Phobia

There are many personality traits that affect social phobia, such as hypersensitive feelings, negative self-image, anticipation of rejection, or inferiority complex, among others. At least 20 percent of those with social disorder have other anxiety problems as well. Social phobias tend to be a lifelong problem, waxing and waning, depending upon the affected person's situation regarding conditions of security and control.

Signs and Symptoms

If you suffer from a social phobia, you may be shy, bashful, timid, and afraid of encounters. A small percentage of people with social phobia also suffer paralyzing fear. You may harbor the emotional anxiety symptoms such as rapid heart rate, muscle tension, and breathlessness triggered when exposed to the feared situation. You may also experience dry mouth, facial flushing, a lump in the throat, and profuse sweating.

The expressions of social phobia are many. Some believe that it is related to fear of public performance. In my practice, I've seen it in an almost blended form that converges with agoraphobia or the abnormal fear of open places. For example, the affected person fears leaving home for social engagements but yet can manage to go to work. When given the option, these people prefer work that does not involve interacting with others.

Diagnosing Social Phobia

Review the following questions to assess your risk for social phobia:

1. Are you fearful that unfamiliar people will over-scrutinize you?
2. Do you worry you will do something accidentally that will humiliate or embarrass you?
3. Do you experience elevated anxiety, near panic, or even full-blown panic when in social situations?
4. Do you avoid social situations to prevent the stress you know you will feel?
5. Do you suffer anticipation anxiety, meaning that just the thought of attending a social event upsets you?
6. Do you worry that others around you will notice that you are nervous?
7. Do you realize your fears and worries are excessive but you find it hard or impossible to ignore them?
8. Are you distressed that you exhibit these fears?

If you answered yes to any of these questions, it's important that you see your doctor and talk openly about your concern. Get an accurate diagnosis, and then talk with your doctor about the natural therapies discussed in my program to see if they might help alleviate your phobias and fears.

AGORAPHOBIA

Another common anxiety disorder affects those who live in fear of being in places or situations that are potentially embarrassing or uncomfortable. The agoraphobic is overly anxious about situations in which she might be entrapped or from which escape is difficult, if not impossible.

Unlike an individual suffering from multiple phobias, the agoraphobic has a cluster of phobias that relate to multiple domains such as transportation or groups of people. If this person is only phobic to people, then the diagnosis of social phobia is more appropriate.

Who's at Risk?

Agoraphobia is a disorder that usually accompanies other anxiety disorders. For instance, statistically, about 95 percent of those with agoraphobia also have panic disorder. More women are afflicted with agoraphobia than men, and it usually flares during their twenties, if coexisting with panic disorder.

In the case of simple agoraphobia, the anxiety reaches the level of panic-like symptoms but never escalates into an actual panic attack. To qualify as a nonpanic form of agoraphobia, the symptoms of panic disorder must not be fully present even though a few of those characteristics are present.

Signs and Symptoms

With agoraphobia, you have emotional or autonomic symptoms that are demonstrations of anxiety whenever you are faced with the feared situation. For example, you might worry about having a panic attack in a public dwelling. Just the thought of the public place can give you anxiety symptoms (see page 31), such as rapid heart rate, difficulty breathing, and even high blood pressure. You might feel helpless, dependent on others, and even depressed if you stay housebound for any length of time. Patients with agoraphobia are usually afraid of travel, crowds, elevators, bridges, and being alone outside.

Some agoraphobics will venture out with the intention of enduring their discomfort. They may deal with it on their own, but such people often prefer to go out with a trusted companion. If agoraphobia did not cause people to become housebound, all of the other symptoms such as avoiding social activities or reduced participation of other significant but personal activities could easily lead to a different diagnosis, or even a group of other disorders such as panic disorder or generalized anxiety disorder.

Diagnosing Agoraphobia

Review the following questions to see if you have signs of agoraphobia:

1. Are you extremely afraid of being trapped in a location you will find hard to leave?
2. Are you afraid of being embarrassed in a situation from which it will be hard to escape?
3. Are you afraid of developing panic-like symptoms or even a panic attack if you leave home?
4. Do you typically become extremely distressed in a crowd or standing in a line of strangers?
5. Do you fear traveling on a train, plane, or bus?
6. Do you require a companion to leave home?
7. Is your travel away from home limited only to your workplace or the grocery store?
8. Are you worried you may suffer diarrhea, dizziness, or other physical symptoms of panic and fear if you leave home?

If you answered yes to any of these questions, talk to your doctor about your concern and seek an accurate diagnosis. There are many therapies discussed in my holistic program that may help you. Discuss these with your doctor to see which ones work best for your situation.

PANIC DISORDER

A panic attack is a single event. However, the diagnosis of a panic disorder requires that the patient have at least two unexpected panic attacks (usually, however, he has many more) before seeking help.

Risk Factors

Panic disorder often runs in families. Findings suggest that if one identical twin has panic disorder, the other twin will also develop panic disorder about 40 percent of the time. It also happens twice as often in women as men, and affects about 2 percent of the general population each year.

Most panic disorder sufferers begin experiencing panic attacks before the age of twenty-five, although it is less likely for these attacks to begin in early childhood. Also, panic disorder rarely develops after age forty-five. Panic attacks can come and go throughout one's life, but there can be years of freedom between series of attacks. Although there are a myriad of pharmaceuticals designed for the treatment of this disease, statistics show that as many as one out of three patients are poorly controlled with these medications.

Panic attacks may and frequently do occur unexpectedly, without having any risk factors or triggering event. However, they can also become situational or related to a phobic object or event. In a true case of panic disorder, the attack must come unexpectedly even though a known object or situation may also trigger it.

In addition to the diagnostic requirement of spontaneity, the patient must also be worried about having another attack. While physical substances such as caffeine or alcohol can trigger panic attacks, the true panic disorder patient will have the attacks without provocation.

There is a major association between bipolar disorder (see pages 34–35) and panic disorder patients. Almost half of the patients with panic disorder may have some level of mood disorder. The depression experienced in a bipolar patient sometimes triggers the beginning of a panic disorder.

Signs and Symptoms

A panic attack takes place within a finite period of time. During the attack, there is a sudden, explosive wave of intense fear and discomfort, which peaks in about ten minutes.

To qualify officially as a panic attack, there must be at least four or more of the following symptoms present during the incident:

- palpitations (pounding or fast heartbeat)
- sweating
- trembling or shaking
- shortness of breath or sensation of smothering
- feelings of choking
- chest pain
- nausea
- dizziness (feeling unsteady, light-headed, or faint)
- fear of losing control
- fear of going crazy
- numbness or tingling
- chills or hot flashes
- feelings of disorientation
- feelings of detachment

I once treated a teenage girl who said she began having panic attacks during early adolescence but told no one because she thought she was going crazy. This young woman was afraid to tell anyone, thinking they might force her into a mental hospital.

The first experience of panic *is* a shock to most people, and they handle it in different ways. Many rush to an emergency room, thinking they are having a heart attack. Others believe they are so oxygen-deprived that they dial 911. The panic attack itself is not limited to any special category of anxiety because it may occur in most forms, including social phobia, specific phobia, post-traumatic stress, acute stress, and agoraphobia.

The frequency of attacks varies among individuals, and even within a particular person's life. The attacks may occur every day for a week and then disappear for several months. Some people experience mini-attacks where they have one or two symptoms, but not the four or more associated with a full-blown attack.

The attacks themselves are bad enough, and the anxiety about future attacks is an additional burden. Nevertheless, there is even more to worry about for the panic disorder patient. Many of them worry that some undiagnosed, life-threatening illness is causing their symptoms. I find it difficult to convince patients that they don't have an underlying heart condition or something even worse.

The panic patient is also overly concerned about the possibility of "going crazy." In my experience, their general anxiety levels rise and fall constantly between attacks. When their anxiety is low, they are logical and understanding of their condition, but when their general anxiety peaks, they question the diagnosis. If they begin an escalating process of avoidance, they have reached the level of a true disability. It gets even worse if the patient begins a frantic search for a brain tumor or other rare disease they are certain they have.

There are many physical manifestations of anxiety and panic that can be easily measured, such as respiration rate, heartbeat, rhythm, skin temperature, and so on, but these measurements only tell us how the body is reacting to the experience, not *why* the event is occurring.

Panic Triggers

A panic trigger is something that sets off the attack, but it is not the pathological mechanism behind the attack. Psychological triggers are probably the most common stimulant for panic attacks. Everyone knows that stress can trigger almost every known physical or psychological dysfunction, including a panic attack. Not far behind are physical triggers, including food sensitivity, hypoglycemia, and fatigue, among others. Some especially sensitive people can even experience panic attacks triggered by exposure to a chemical agent, for example, such as slightly elevated carbon dioxide (CO_2) levels in the blood. I will give you some natural therapies for panic attacks later in the book (see Step 2).

Specific Forms of Panic

Along with the panic attacks that result from certain stressors or physical triggers, there are other forms of panic that might occur.

Pulmonary panic. It's long been suspected that people with lung (pulmonary) problems have a higher incidence of panic than the general population. In findings published in the May

2002 issue of the journal *Psychiatry Research*, researchers reported in a study of forty-five asthma patients that 52 percent had at least one current anxiety problem. Overall, 60 percent of all patients said they had depression, anxiety, or both.

Nocturnal panic. One out of four people with panic disorder experiences nocturnal panic attacks. A sleeping person will awaken in a full state of panic. The frequency of an attack can be monthly, weekly, or even several times nightly. Usually the symptoms include rapid heartbeat, shortness of breath, and a profound sense of fear, which is an acute state of sympathetic nervous system arousal. However, this sympathetic arousal is triggered more by physical phenomena (such as acidity or hypoglycemia) than it is a response to a psychological component.

Nocturnal panic is not a nightmare, nor is it a night terror, which tends to occur in stage 4 sleep, nor is it related to sleep apnea or REM sleep. It is not a seizure or related to any abnormal EEG pattern. More commonly, it occurs a little over an hour after one falls asleep, during the passage through stage 2 or stage 3 sleep.

Diagnosing Panic Disorder

Review the following to see if you have symptoms of panic disorder:

1. Do you experience sudden attacks of intense fear and discomfort?
2. During the attack do you experience any of the following?
   * a pounding or fast heartbeat
   * shortness of breath

- a chest pain that feels like a heart attack
- a faint, unsteady feeling as if you might pass out
- a feeling as if everything around you is unreal
- a feeling as if you are out of control
- a feeling as if you are going crazy
- a feeling as if you might die
- a feeling of tingling or numbness anywhere on the body
- wanting to run away from where you are

If you have any of these signs or symptoms, talk to your doctor and seek an accurate diagnosis. Then consider the natural therapies discussed in my holistic program to see if they might work for your panic disorder.

OBSESSIVE-COMPULSIVE DISORDER (OCD)

Obsessive-compulsive disorder (OCD) is yet one more anxiety disorder. Persons with OCD have persistent and recurring thoughts, impulses, and images that are intrusive and often inappropriate, all which create great internal anxiety and distress. These obsessive thoughts, impulses, and images are not simple worries about everyday problems. Rather, the symptoms are so intense that they force you to exert considerable effort in order to return to normal thought. Within time, the person affected with OCD comes to know, sooner or later, that these imposing forces are not helpful or normal.

In the past it was thought that OCD symptoms were meant to alleviate an underlying anxiety and that any attempt to resist the anxiety would force the patient back to habitual actions. But some new studies suggest that there is hyperactivity in an area in the front part of the brain called the anterior cingulate cortex.

No one, yet, can explain exactly why this exaggerated activity occurs in those with OCD, but electrophysiological and brain scan evidence supports this concept. This specific circuit monitors other thoughts, scanning for errors and generating error signals to the higher levels of the brain. By error, I mean that a current experience has come in conflict with the person's standards or goals. When the system of the brain that exerts top-down control is alerted, it tries to resolve the conflict. Everyone has this type of circuit, but in OCD patients, this system is vastly over-critical.

OCD complicates the treatment of the other problems because there is no completely satisfactory drug of choice for OCD. Many drugs such as the tricyclic antidepressants, monoamine oxidase inhibitors, neuroleptics, and benzodiazepines, among others, have been tried but without good results.

Risk Factors

Unlike some of the other forms of anxiety such as panic disorder or agoraphobia, where females dominate the patient list, OCD occurs more frequently in males. The illness can begin as early as age six, but usually begins in adolescence and early adulthood. Fifteen percent of the patients progressively deteriorate into complete loss of self-sufficiency. On the other end, 5 percent have relatively few symptoms that come and go. All of the others fall somewhere in between. The rate for OCD in immediate family members is much higher than has been recorded for the general population.

OCD frequently coexists with other conditions such as

panic disorder. Another commonly related disorder is hypochondriasis. In fact, hypochondriasis, panic disorder, and OCD frequently occur together. OCD, unipolar depression, and schizophrenia appear to share similar disturbances in the front lobe of the brain.

Some scientists believe that OCD is a response to a streptococcal infection. Although antibiotics have not proved helpful in treating OCD symptoms, it appears that intravenous immunoglobulin therapy has been successful in some patients.

Signs and Symptoms

The OCD patient's obsessive thoughts, impulses, and images are not simple worries. It requires considerable effort to return to normal thought. The compulsive aspect is physical and involves repetitive behaviors such as frequently brushing one's teeth, hoarding behaviors, hair pulling, or double-checking everything repeatedly. It can also take the form of continuous prayer, word repetition or counting, or excessive worry over physical imperfections. It may further manifest itself in the endless rehashing of one particular topic.

A further aspect of this disorder is that the actions are time-consuming. If they occur even one hour a day, they can significantly interfere with a person's normal routine, work, or social relationships. This disorder can further dominate the personality by converting into an eating disorder, trichotillomania (hair pulling), body dysmorphic ideation (concern over an unacceptable body), and hypochondria. When hypochondriacs fail to have any insight into their problem, it means they have reached the delusional level.

The major problem with OCD is its anxiety component is subterranean, that is, the symptoms are meant to alleviate the unfelt underlying anxiety. Any attempt to resist these activities unleashes its power, which then sends the person racing back toward the safety of their habitual actions. Most patients stop trying to resist the habits and form an uncomfortable alliance with their compulsions, trying to accommodate them into their life in whatever way they can.

Once again, although the obsessive-compulsive symptoms may dominate this disorder, there are usually different levels of other forms of anxiety present as well. For example, phobias, panic, social fears, and a basketful of other anxiety-related problems all exist simultaneously with the obsessive-compulsive aspects.

The electrical activity of the nervous system is also involved. When a triggering event is initiated in a laboratory to cause an obsessive symptom, increased autonomic nervous system activity has been recorded. If the patient responds with a compulsive activity, then the physiological excitement in the nervous system is significantly reduced.

There are no laboratory tests that can aid in the diagnosis of OCD, but serotonin-enhancing drugs might make OCD symptoms worse, possibly indicating that excessive serotonin may be a factor in this illness. To the exact contrary, there are findings indicating that moderate to higher doses of paroxetine (a serotonin-enhancing drug) is effective in treating acute symptoms, and decreasing the rate of relapse. It is not unusual for scientific studies to contradict each other. In this case, the contradiction further confirms that OCD and other difficult-to-treat diseases are still baffling to scientists.

Diagnosing Obsessive-Compulsive Disorder

Review the following questions to assess your risk for OCD:

1. Do you suffer persistent, recurring negative thoughts or images?
2. Do these thoughts or images frequently block out other current thoughts?
3. Do you find it almost impossible to ignore or suppress these thoughts and images?
4. Are you aware that these thoughts and images are self-generated and not placed there by others?
5. Do you count everything?
6. Do you repeat words or say phrases under your breath?
7. Are you always pulling your hair or picking your skin?
8. Do you tend to follow rules to the extreme?
9. Do you constantly plan and over-organize?
10. Do you feel guilt more often than anxiety?
11. Do you recognize that your behavior is extreme?

If you answered yes to any of these questions, you may have obsessive-compulsive disorder. Talk to your doctor and seek an accurate diagnosis. Then consider the natural therapies discussed in my holistic program.

Chapter 3

❧

Stress and Adjustment Disorders

"The feeling seems to come out of nowhere, and suddenly my heart rate is pounding in high gear, my head is throbbing, and I can barely catch my breath." While Luke's symptoms were not life-threatening, they are a common reaction to daily stress.

Stress. We all live with it from day to day. Whether from an argument with your spouse, conflict with a co-worker, or living with chronic pain, stress is here to stay. Everyone knows what stress is and yet there are seemingly endless definitions of it. Simply stated, stress describes the various demands and pressures that all of us experience each day. The word "stress" can describe both the stressful situation or stressor, and the symptoms that are experienced, or stress response.

Every situation in our lives, whether positive or negative, causes some response within our psyche and our body. The level of stress response often depends on the suddenness and the degree of threat to our physical and psychological integrity.

"Stress has taken over my life," fifty-one-year-old Diane said. "In one week, my daughter was in a car accident, my husband was laid off, and my sister had a breast biopsy that was positive. What else can I handle? I'm afraid to get out of bed for fear another tragedy will happen."

While normal daily stressors require little in the way of adapting on our part, pathological stress forces us into mobilizing our best defenses and challenges our capacity to cope. How each of us acts under severe pathological stress is dramatically different. Some rise to the occasion and are even motivated by it; others develop anxiety disorders.

GOOD STRESS—BAD STRESS

Most of us interpret stress as negative, but it is not always bad. Buying a home, starting a new job, or having a baby are all positive (called eustress) and reasons to celebrate. Yet all can cause great stress.

What is considered stress to one person may be a source of pleasure to another; it all depends on the person and the source of the stress. For example, your best friend may jump out of an airplane as a member of a skydiving club. For her, this is a positive experience and constitutes a form of emotional excitement. You, however, may respond to just the sound of airplanes taking off and landing with great anxiety.

While the environmental trigger is identical, we all perceive situations in different ways. You may achieve all the emotional excitement you need by watching a suspenseful video in the safety of your home. Your friend may have a very high threshold for emotional excitement and achieve it by jumping off cranes with bungee cords around her ankles or by participating in other dangerous sports. Your threshold for responding to stress is dictated largely by your genetic blueprint.

When we are exposed to a situation perceived as threatening, our bodies prepare for confrontation. The response called fight-or-flight is physical and is controlled by our hormones and nervous system. We are prepared to fight or flee our stressor. Even though we don't live in the age of fighting wild animals, these wild animals exist in such forms as conflict at work or home, traffic jams, a telephone that never stops ringing, and long lines, among others.

If you encounter sufficient stress, it can be measured physically. For example, during stress, blood levels of glucocorticoids, hormones that are generated in the adrenal gland, become elevated. Ironically, these same glucocorticoids are raised during a pleasurable activity like eating or sex. The physical signs of stress, unfortunately, do not tell us whether it is a pleasurable stress or a painful one.

Most authors in the field of psychology now use the words "stress" and "anxiety" interchangeably simply because it is difficult to find a difference in this context. Even when the source of the stress is positive stress, such as the anxiety one feels before receiving a reward or a public recognition, the nervousness still seems to be identical.

A physiologist would argue that there are more measurable (physical) limitations related to stress than there are to anxiety. Yet the studies related to the pathochemistry of anxiety are quite extensive, too, making anxiety equally physical.

Physical and Emotional Responses

We all respond differently to stress. In fact, stress influences males differently than it does females. For instance, one of the heaviest stressors males face in their daily life is failure or defeat; females in our society are most stressed by social instability. Whatever the stressful situation is, from a business meeting to a personal or work deadline to coping with active kids, the physical response still occurs. The symptoms of stress, listed below, can vary in intensity but will predictably happen during stressful moments.

Empirical studies confirm that a strong sense of control is vital for our health and stability. Likewise, the level of stress felt (your stress response) is directly related to the level of control available. Curiously, the same is true if you feel the stress is predictable. Regardless of the internal knowledge of control or predictability, the physical signs such as hypervigilance, excitability, and apprehension will still be present to the same degree. For the stress to be negative, the experience must be perceived as harmful, something to be avoided or at least reduced. The stress must also cause a heightened physical state such as restlessness or emotional volatility, as well as overreacting to events. This state must be married to the fear of something being in jeopardy: finances, relationships, job security, health.

Common Stress Reactions

- anger
- anxiety
- apathy
- back pain
- chest pain or tightness
- colitis
- depression
- headaches
- heart palpitations
- hives
- impotence

- inability to concentrate
- inability to relax
- irregular menstrual periods
- irritable bowel syndrome (IBS)
- jaw pain
- lack of energy
- loss of sexual desire
- mood swings
- neck pain
- rapid pulse
- rashes
- short temper
- short-term memory loss
- sleep disorders
- weight gain
- weight loss

The Fear Circuit

It's generally accepted that anyone with an anxiety or stress disorder is biologically vulnerable, and life experiences may accentuate or diminish this tendency. The exact physiological pathologies are yet to be determined, but we do have answers to large pieces of the puzzle. First, the affected person's brain is believed to have an overactive alarm system, and this sensitivity can range from slightly vulnerable to severely vulnerable.

Just beneath the main mass of the brain is an area called the amygdala, the control tower for all acute emotions, including fear and anxiety. The amygdala draws information from and passes data to other powerful centers in the brain such as the frontal lobe, the brain stem (locus ceruleus), the thalamus and hippocampus, and the cortical processing areas. The frontal lobe keeps the entire system hypervigilant for danger by overreacting and distorting what it sees and hears. In many people, the frontal lobe is full of catastrophic thoughts and pessimistic evaluations. Scientists postulate that poor or even complete miscoordination of information between all of these brain centers may cause the amygdala to overreact, thus producing a panic attack or exaggerated stress response.

The amygdala sits inside a larger area called the limbic system (page 29), which includes the hippocampus (this center helps to put a little reality back into the fear). The limbic system generates all emotions, which have incredible power to move people to action. A thought without an emotion behind it is empty because thoughts do not draw energy. Emotions pull enormous volumes of measurable energy toward them.

When fears get going, they influence massive neurological areas of the brain and a substantial number of chemicals, especially brain neurotransmitters (see pages 83–88). These negative emotions do all the damage because they have enormous power, a virtual tornado of fear and anxiety that is completely unforgettable. A fearful thought without an attached emotion is not taken seriously by anyone, including your own mind and body.

ACUTE STRESS REACTION

It's no news that we live in a world full of stresses. Each day, our bodies and minds can be compromised by disease as well as natural and man-made disasters. With traumatic events, some people rise to the challenge and react with determination and persistence. Yet others are overwhelmed by life's major stressors and lose all confidence in their ability to cope. Before we discuss how to resolve stress-related problems, it's important to define several categories of stress.

Immediately after a traumatic event, people often manifest a pattern of anxiety symptoms and cognitive disturbances referred to frequently as an acute stress reaction. The symptoms of acute stress reaction begin within minutes of the traumatic event and disappear within days (even hours). This reaction is an adaptation of the mind and body to manage the painful thoughts and feelings associated with the event, so that those afflicted can go on with their lives, even if minimally.

Signs and Symptoms

With acute stress reaction, you may feel a state of numbness or shock, reduced attention span, agitation, disorientation, withdrawal, difficulty sleeping, or the other anxiety symptoms listed on page 31. These symptoms usually disappear in a few days after the traumatic experience.

After forty-six-year-old Kit gave me a rundown of her typical day, it was apparent why she was experiencing insomnia, rapid heart rate, and shortness of breath—her anxiety level was off the chart.

Every day, Kit gets up at 4:30 A.M. to make school lunches for her three children and do other household chores. Employed full-time as a paralegal, she often works without taking a break or even eating lunch. Three days a week, she helps coach the swim team at her oldest son's school. She also assists with her daughter's soccer league, helping to do the weekly newsletter. It is usually 7:00 P.M. before Kit finishes her last after-school carpool and gets home to greet her husband and start dinner. After dinner, she does the dishes, pays the bills, monitors homework, and more.

Is it any wonder that when Kit's brother was killed suddenly in an automobile accident, she was so distressed that she had to be hospitalized for a short period? While Kit had it all—family, career, commitments—she, like so many of my patients, simply did not have enough energy to take care of her own mental health. She had pushed herself beyond reasonable limits and when the acute stress occurred, she had no energy to cope with the loss.

I explained to Kit that stress levels measured among working mothers sometimes approach the levels of those in combat. Single working women and women who are single parents, juggling kids and career, are often greatly stressed. With natural supplements and some lifestyle changes, including backing off some commitments, Kit was able to recover from the acute stress and regain some control over her busy life.

Factors to Consider

Usually the diagnosis of acute stress reaction is made immediately after a stressful situation if there has been a significant emotional reaction to the event. Herein lies the key: This diagnosis is only good for one month. If symptoms continue past one month, the diagnosis changes to the more serious post-traumatic stress disorder (PTSD), discussed on pages 66–71. During this period, the doctors involved in the diagnosis will determine if any physical damage has occurred. A physical cause for the symptoms must be ruled out before a psychiatric diagnosis is appropriate.

Diagnosing Acute Stress Reaction

Review the following questions to see if you might have acute stress reaction:

1. Were you exposed to an event within the last thirty days that could have resulted in your death or serious injury? (If this has exceeded thirty days, then you may be included in the PTSD category.)
2. Were you exposed to a traumatic event within the past thirty days that could have resulted in death or serious injury to others around you?
3. Did you feel helpless, lacking control?
4. Have you been reliving this event in your thoughts or dreams, including daydreams?

If you answered yes to any of these questions, you may be experiencing an acute stress reaction. Call your doctor and get an accurate diagnosis. Also, discuss using the natural therapies discussed in my holistic program to revitalize your body's energy and calm the anxiety.

ADJUSTMENT DISORDER

Emotional or behavioral symptoms that occur because of a significant and stressful change in circumstances such as divorce or moving from one region of the country to another can be attributed to adjustment disorders. The diagnosis depends on the amount of social or work impairment because of the reaction to the stressors. Relatively common but stressful events underlie this problem rather than the horrific trauma that causes post-traumatic stress disorder. Nevertheless, the reaction to the change can be extreme, causing significant depression, maladaptive conduct, and even attempts at suicide or homicide. This type of anxiety disorder is common and frequently goes without treatment. The most severe responses to unexpected and sudden changes occur in those who already have unstable personalities; they just cannot adapt.

Personality is another consideration with adjustment disorder. It is usually someone with a personality disorder who suffers most from sudden change such as the loss of a job or a relationship. Failure to adjust can precipitate sudden, explosive reactions.

Twenty-seven-year-old Marissa suffered with adjustment disorder when she moved to California from her small town in the Midwest. Although she had a history of attention deficit disorder (ADD) and anxiety, she did not think it would hinder her in finding a job and making friends. Yet after being hired—and fired—three times in seven months, Marissa simply could not function. Her self-confidence deteriorated to the point where she hated to answer the phone or open her mail for fear it was yet another rejection. Her boyfriend abruptly ended their relationship because of her paranoia and nervousness, and she lost her car when she stopped making payments.

When I first saw Marissa, she said she slept only a few hours each night because her mind was on "red alert," ruminating about all her failures and fears. I suggested that Marissa take 5-HTP (pages 160–161) to help calm her, along with tyrosine (page 158), which generates the neurotransmitter dopamine. She also started taking the natural sleep formula Body Enhancer to increase healing sleep (see page 227 and Resources). Within a few weeks, Marissa had reversed her downhill spiral and was sleeping more than seven hours a night and waking up feeling refreshed. She landed a teaching position at a private school and found a roommate with an apartment near the coast. Marissa finally regained her energy, focus, and productivity and felt as if there was no problem too big for her to handle.

Signs and Symptoms

While anxiety and depression are the two most common symptoms of adjustment disorder, unexpected behavioral changes are frequent, including truancy, vandalism, reckless driving, fighting, and defaulting on debts. When a worker with a severe personality disorder is suddenly fired from a job, he may return to the workplace and take it out on others. (An extreme example of this behavior would be what we now call "going postal.")

Factors to Consider

The diagnosis of adjustment disorder is almost always secondary to other forms of mental instability such as bipolar disorder, paranoid personality disorder, mood disorder, and obsessive-compulsive disorder, among others.

Diagnosing Adjustment Disorder

Review the following questions to see if you might have adjustment disorder:

1. Have you suffered a significant stress within the last three months?
2. Is your suffering so great that you don't seem to be getting over it?

3. Are these stressful feelings interfering with your job or social life?
4. Are these stressful feelings causing you sleepless nights?
5. Do you suspect the emotional pain will not go away without professional help?

If you answered yes to any of these questions, talk to your doctor about issues and symptoms associated with the adjustment disorder and get an accurate diagnosis. Then talk with your doctor about using some of the natural therapies discussed in my holistic program.

POST-TRAUMATIC STRESS DISORDER (PTSD)

Post-traumatic stress disorder is the most severe reaction to stress humans can suffer. People with PTSD have experienced or witnessed an event or series of events that were life-threatening or a threat to their own or others' physical integrity. In the midst of this event, the affected person's response was intense fear, a sense of helplessness, or horror.

With PTSD, the stress is so severe that it tests the limits of a person's mental and physical survivability. Witnessing or being a part of an event that is life-threatening or that threatens to severely damage a person, especially when there is absolute helplessness, is almost unbearable. The intense sense of helplessness and horror cannot help but shake the foundations of any prior internal stability. Most of the time the PTSD patient relives the event through distressing and intrusive images, thoughts about the awful event, dreams that resemble the fearful situation, and frightening flashbacks.

Signs and Symptoms

Following a traumatic event, the person may experience one or more of the following symptoms: frequent distressing and intrusive images, thoughts or perceptions of the original event, a series of frightening dreams with or without the images of the event, distress when exposed to cues that symbolize or resemble the fearful situation, and traumatic flashbacks.

For some with PTSD, there is a tendency to avoid anything that is associated with the trauma: conversations, persons, places, or feelings connected to the trauma. Some people cope by detaching themselves from all feelings. Others do the opposite and fill themselves with intense feelings of anger or depression.

Some PTSD patients may develop partial amnesia or feelings of detachment, or they may restrict their range of feelings altogether. Often they begin making negative predictions regarding their work, family, and life span. The person may also have sleep difficulties, sudden anger, poor concentration, hypervigilance, or she may overreact when startled. Usually these symptoms begin within a month of the event. However, along with the reliving of the experience, the person often suffers a constant mix of guilt, anxiety, anhedonia (deriving no current pleasure from a previously pleasurable thought or activity).

Factors to Consider

The first two days after the event the anxiety felt can be labeled acute stress reaction (page 60). But if the symptoms continue past four weeks, the diagnosis is changed to PTSD. Any extremely traumatic stress can precipitate this disorder in almost any normal person. However, in an individual with a preexisting mental problem, PTSD is usually triggered by an event that would barely faze a more stable personality. For example, if you currently suffer with anxiety and phobias, your chance of having PTSD is far greater than someone who does not have these mental disorders.

Epidemiological studies conducted at the University of Modena in Italy and published in a 2001 issue of the journal *Neuropsychobiology* indicate that PTSD is clearly becoming a major health concern worldwide. This problem affects occupational and social capabilities of a substantial number of people. The authors of this particular study suggest that PTSD generates a dysregulation in the neurotransmitter (a brain chemical) and sympathetic nervous systems, discussed on page 49. In this Italian study, researchers suggest that antidepressant drugs may be the best therapeutic response for PTSD. The reason for this choice of drugs is that they also are effective for depression, panic disorder, and social anxiety, which are commonly found along with PTSD. Antidepressant drugs therefore cover therapeutically a large area of mental distress.

According to other findings published in 1997 in the *Journal of Clinical Psychiatry*, 80 percent of those with PTSD meet the criteria for at least one other psychiatric disorder and a sizable number have more than one. While the additional mental problems may have been the result of the original stress, there are numerous studies that indicate they were already present before the stress and materially contributed to the severity of trauma as a result of the stress. This also affects the prognosis for successful recovery.

Other factors to consider:

PTSD can destroy brain tissue. Stress has definite detrimental effects on the brain. For example, it can deter growth of neurons. The part of the brain called the hippocampus has been found to be important to learning and memory. However, those with PTSD have been found to have a reduced volume of mass in the hippocampus compared to that of the average person. In fact, people who have suffered PTSD have had memory loss as high as 35 percent. Combat veterans and people who have suffered child abuse may have as much as a 40 percent reduction in hippocampal size.

Still, there is a group that believes that the people who suffer the most from PTSD are those who possessed an undersized hippocampal area *prior* to the traumatic stress. These experts believe that the smaller organ is a result of their genetic makeup, which makes these people far less resilient and more vulnerable to the impact of stress.

PTSD changes body chemistry. Traumatic stress may or may not include direct physical damage. Nevertheless, there is a severe internal shock to the body's metabolism. When applied to physical diseases, severe stress means changes in chemistry, physiology, and the functionality of tissues, and all of these changes are measurable.

A very important change has to do with the internal and external assault by free radicals. These are highly reactive and unstable molecules produced by the body that can disrupt and tear apart vital cell structures. Free radicals are destructive to every part of the neurological system. While free radicals have been widely accepted as a major cause for physical disease, they are increasingly being connected to mental disease as well.

PTSD imprints brain cells. Traumatic fear burrows down in every direction like roots on a tree, spreading to every nook and cranny in the brain, seeking nourishment. Anxiety-generating thoughts and images go everywhere, crossing all boundaries; no place is overlooked. It is as though the fearful emotions permanently stain or tattoo the affected cells so they will never forget the incident.

Fear tends to generalize in the brain, spreading out to multiple cerebral systems. One of the latest revelations is that learned fear, the core of anxiety, is not obliterated by erasing the original learning but by blocking the learning that is already instilled in the brain. In other words, you don't have the choice of destroying your memory; your brain doesn't have a program or method of doing that. Instead, you must learn to consciously block what you have learned.

Survival is the supreme goal of any animal. It makes sense then that learning what to fear is easy, but purging it from your mind later is almost impossible. The body has set it up this way for survival and made it an immutable system. Unfortunately, the brain cannot use the same generalizing process to remove or extinguish the fear. We simply cannot get traumatic memories out as easily as they come into our minds.

Diagnosing Post-Traumatic Stress Disorder

Consider the following questions to see if you might have post-traumatic stress disorder:

1. Were you exposed to a traumatic event that could have resulted in your death or serious injury?
2. Were you exposed to a traumatic event that could have resulted in death or serious injury to others around you?
3. Did you feel helpless, lacking any control?
4. Have you been reliving this event in your thoughts or dreams, including daydreams?
5. Do recurring distressing recollections of the event continually intrude into your thoughts?

6. Are you experiencing frightening dreams that may or may not accurately reflect the event?
7. Do you find yourself reliving the experience through flashbacks, hallucinations, images, or illusions?
8. Do events or activities around you that symbolize the event trigger the distress?
9. Do you find it impossible to avoid thoughts, feelings, or conversations associated with the trauma?
10. Do you have amnesia for various parts of the trauma?
11. Have you lost interest in many of your pre-traumatic activities?
12. Do you feel detached and distant from others?
13. Are you negative about your future?
14. Do you have trouble sleeping?
15. Do angry outbursts come easily?
16. Is it difficult to concentrate?
17. Is your present state of mental health adversely affecting your job, family, or social life?

If you answered yes to any of these questions, call your doctor to see if you have post-traumatic stress disorder. Get an accurate diagnosis and then consider the natural therapies discussed in my holistic program.

HELP IS AVAILABLE

So, when do you need to seek help for anxiety and stress disorders? It's really up to you and how these disorders are robbing your quality of life. I ask my patients the following questions:

1. Are the painful symptoms of your experience not declining steadily as time passes?
2. Do you suffer with disrupted sleep with no way to restore your natural sleep patterns?
3. Do current stressful events aggravate the old wound?

If you answered yes to these questions, know that there is hope. You can find a host of answers to your stress-related problem in my 5-step program. First get a proper diagnosis and then talk with your doctor about using some of the natural therapies discussed in my holistic program.

Chapter 4

Finding Natural Relief

When fifty-one-year-old Joan came to my clinic, she was so distraught that she could barely fill out the patient information forms. This mother of two young adult children had been married for thirty years, in what she thought was a perfect relationship . . . until the day her husband invited her out for dinner and told her he was leaving that night for another woman. Joan's husband admitted that he could no longer tolerate her high anxiety, fearful nature, and over-controlling behavior; he was in love with another woman, and he wanted out.

Joan was shocked. She immediately depersonalized, which means to mentally remove herself from reality as an outsider looking in, and thought she was having a nightmare. She wasn't. The next week, Joan packed her belongings and went to California to stay with her mother.

After talking at length with Joan, I suggested that she try some natural therapies to ease the anxiety and fears, so she could take care of the business at hand. I put her on my daily B vitamin injections and asked her to take a magnesium cap-

sule, 300 milligrams three times a day. Joan knew she had to
see a divorce lawyer and wanted to meet with her mother's pas-
tor for counseling. I expected the vitamin injections would
give her the energy she needed to move on with a plan and
enough relief to unbind her from the crippling acute or sudden anxiety.

Because Joan had a lengthy history of disturbed sleep, I
had her take the Body Enhancer natural sleep remedy (see Resources) and eliminate this problem as a drain on her energy.
As soon as we broke through her emotional paralysis, her natural good sense took over. Joan was able to stand up for herself
and fight back. It was not long after that she got in control of
the situation, and her husband agreed to relinquish the family
house and a large sum of money to Joan. She moved back to
her hometown and continued the natural therapies, adjusting
the doses now and then. The last I heard, Joan had remarried
and was volunteering at several nonprofit agencies. Joan is just
one of many patients with anxiety who have benefited from
natural therapies.

Twenty-nine-year-old Eric found that alternative treatments gave him a feeling of confidence and control—when
medications had failed. This young man was very intelligent
yet had never pursued college because of lack of funding. He
enlisted in the army after high school but, following a stressful
incident, he attempted suicide and was released.

Eric found a job in the local library that allowed him to use
his sharp mind on the telephone with patrons. He seemed to
be leveling out until his roommate was killed in a car accident.
Eric then became completely incapacitated and developed sur-
vivor guilt, panic, and agoraphobia, which caused him to co-
coon in his apartment, avoiding contact with anyone.

Completely opposed to taking medications, Eric was in a

handicapped situation until he came to my clinic. After taking his personal history, I started Eric on a simple multivitamin with kelp and a calcium-magnesium supplement, three times a day. I had him take 50 milligrams of 5-HTP, twice daily, to ease anxiety, and suggested that he take a natural sleep supplement (Body Enhancer) at bedtime to help provide restful sleep. Eric also began to exercise daily at his apartment building's fitness center and he changed his diet by adding more complex carbohydrates and eating small frequent meals rather than two or three large ones to keep his energy level high.

Within weeks, this young man went from being depressed and neurotic to actually smiling at strangers on the city bus. Today, Eric continues these basic alternative therapies and has enrolled in a community college to study software programming. He even has a girlfriend—for the first time in his life.

MY APPROACH: GET BACK TO NATURE

My 5-step holistic program is filled with easy, workable solutions—natural therapies and lifestyle habits—that you can start immediately as you finally get relief from mild anxiety. If used appropriately, this multifaceted program can boost self-efficacy, and we doctors know that feeling in control of your health is essential for wellness. These natural interventions might allow you to take less medication, have fewer laboratory tests and doctor visits, and, most importantly, be an active participant in self-care. If a natural therapy has proven safe and effective for 4,000 years, then who am I to question it!

The chances are that you are busy and want answers—fast—on how to ease mild anxiety so you can continue being active and productive. That's why I organized this book in an easy-to-read format. After reading about how to get an accurate diagnosis with Step 1, you will move on to Steps 2 to 5 and learn about natural supplements to ease anxiety, specific nutrients to keep your body chemicals balanced, easy lifestyle habits to get calming sleep, and why exercise is vital to de-stress.

While there are medications that work to ease anxiety symptoms, I agree with those integrative medicine experts who believe herbs and other alternative therapies may have a *milder effect* at doing the same—*but without the adverse side effects of pharmaceuticals and outrageous cost.* For instance, journal studies confirm that the herb peppermint is effective in relieving post-operative nausea in patients and costs just pennies compared to pharmaceuticals. I've found through clinical trials that peppermint also eases anxiety and obsessive worrying in those who have panic attacks. Valerian, a bitter herb, has superb sedative properties that can be used to calm the central nervous system, making it useful for treating anxiety, insomnia, and stress at just pennies a dose. When used correctly, this over-the-counter herbal remedy is safe, effective, and works for millions of men and women.

To help you understand my natural treatment program for easing anxiety disorders, I need to first explain how conventional medical and psychological treatment techniques work. These techniques recognize two main approaches:

1. Cognitive-behavioral and related talk therapies; and
2. Pharmaceutical (drug) therapy.

Talk Therapy

Talk therapy is the classical treatment emanating from Freud and peers. Freud was instrumental in organizing and initiating specific treatments, which gave legitimacy to anxiety as a disease and brought some science into an otherwise baffling field.

The analytical approach. The theory behind the analytical approach (with the patient on a couch), assumes there are deep-rooted intrapsychic conflicts between Freud's structural model of the id, the ego, and the superego that usually stem from childhood. These early conflicts must be recovered from repressed memories so the patient can develop insight into the origin of the problem. The new insight, it is thought, will cause remission of symptoms.

Analytical psychotherapy is gradually being phased out by younger, drug-oriented psychiatrists and has lost ground mainly because it requires years of additional training, the training is costly, and it takes years to create change in the patient (if at all). It is also extremely expensive for the patient.

Pavlov's conditioned reflex. Ivan Pavlov, a Russian scientist, introduced a new term into psychiatric jargon: conditioned reflex. His experiments with dogs proved that an animal's nervous system could be trained to react to a triggering object or situation, suggesting, for instance, danger to the animal even after the danger has passed. This greatly expanded the possible causes for mental illness and opened up a measurable approach.

Nondirective psychotherapy. This type of therapy is based on a person-to-person relationship between the counselor and the client. The emphasis is on the here-and-now and the client is encouraged to open up with a free flow of thoughts. In many ways the client leads the therapy, as he reacts openly and determines the course of conversation.

Cognitive-behavioral therapy. This type of talk therapy attempts to change the thoughts and behaviors that generate psychological symptoms. A number of specific techniques are used such as cognitive restructuring or self-statements for self-control and to aid in coping and stopping certain thoughts. The techniques described below are also under this umbrella.

Exposure therapy. With exposure therapy, the affected person confronts the feared object or situation. As you might imagine, this type of therapy is most often used in cases of simple phobias. Typically, this treatment is well structured and supervised so it is safe for the patient. The treatment must be repeated frequently to be successful.

Imaginal exposure therapy. While basically the same as exposure therapy, imaginal exposure therapy takes place in the mind. The feared object or situation is only imagined, not confronted. The therapist directs the patient as she envisions the feared object to maintain safe control over the anxiety experienced.

Relaxation training. The idea here is to learn how to relax all the muscles of the body and then to use this new anxiety control technique during exposure to the feared situation or object. The confrontational sessions are usually increasingly difficult.

Breathing retraining. Here the breath rather than muscles are used to help the person relax. Patients are taught to control diaphragmatic breathing and perhaps to combine it with some special medication when anxious.

Biofeedback. The goal is to learn how to relax the blood vessels so that they dilate and warm the body. The warmth relaxes the muscles and reduces anxiety. As with the other techniques, biofeedback also demonstrates to the anxious patient that they are still in control, which is very reassuring.

Supportive counseling and group therapy. With counseling, the patient gets a sense of support, safety, and encouragement. In individual counseling or in a group, patients may vent their feelings, test out their thoughts and plans with others, and see that they are not the only ones with these kinds of problems. The focus is on current, real-life problems, with little emphasis on childhood experiences.

Self-help groups. These are educational platforms where the focus is on new drugs or techniques for professional help or self-help. Often there are suggestions regarding diet and nutritional supplements that relate to the focus of each self-help group.

Exposure and response prevention. Used to treat obsessive-compulsive disorder (pages 50–54), the patient is exposed to a specific trigger and then prevented from engaging in that obsessive-compulsive act. For example, the hands of the patient are dirtied, and he is then prevented from washing them. This is identical to exposure therapy except that the focus is on a behavior rather than a trigger object or situation.

Other psychological techniques. Other techniques, including hypnosis, are used during talk therapy.

All of these forms just described have taken a backseat to drugs. If you've barely even heard of some of these therapies, it's because many have never become popular, even though most of them have been available since the 1950s.

In theory, these techniques are successful in treating anxiety. Under proper management and with a talented therapist, they can work. However, sometimes the therapy programs are often loosely planned and the therapists are poorly trained. A large health care service center may need to list the program as one of their services in order to receive accreditation or funding, but, in fact, the program exists in name only.

A great deal of the change has come about because of a shift in the government's attitude toward health care. By allowing big business to create managed health care systems such as HMOs and PPOs and by providing some of the care itself, the government has insisted on a system where speed, simplicity, and low cost are the standard and quality is negotiable.

Drug Therapy

It's no secret that drugs are the fastest treatment approach around, so they jump to the top of the list when it comes to treating anxiety disorders. Primary care physicians can write prescriptions for psychiatric problems and that eliminates the cost of a specialist. Like any business today, psychiatry is all about time and money. Just as the old-fashioned family doctor has been replaced by the nurse practitioner or the physician's assistant, psychotherapy has been relegated to the status of an add-on therapy, but only if the patient insists on it and can afford it.

Commonly used medications. Let's briefly review the drugs commonly used in the treatment of anxiety, phobias, and panic disorder. I discussed the tranquilizing benzodiazepines such as Valium (diazepam) and Xanax (alprazolam) on page 13. The selective serotonin reuptake inhibitors (SSRIs) are a widely used group of antidepressants, including drugs such as Prozac (fluoxetine) and Zoloft (sertraline), frequently prescribed for anxiety, panic disorder, obsessive-compulsive disorder, and social phobia. Anticonvulsants such as Klonopin (clonazepam) and Topamax (topiramate) are also prescribed for anxiety disorders. Because new drugs for anxiety are appearing all the time, it is not useful to mention any more than a representative sampling.

While drug therapy can be effective, it's important to note that medications are chemicals normally not found in human tissue. As described on pages 10–16, if taken improperly, these foreign chemicals are potent and therefore hazardous to human health. Drugs may pose health risks even if taken properly. While the risk is not high, it is still there. Upon closer inspection of drugs, there are actually multiple risks depending upon the number of known side effects.

With benefits come risks. With many of these drugs, patients risk both short-term and long-term negative effects. Short-term adverse effects include headaches or nausea, while long-term risks involve the liver, blood pressure, and other body organs or systems. Patients also risk semipermanent or permanent neurochemical changes that may leave them with post-medication problems (see pages 15–16). In other words, when you discontinue an anti-anxiety agent or other drug, you could have post-withdrawal symptoms that will last for months or even years.

If drugs did not possess a toxic potential, then a doctor's prescription would not be necessary. Your doctor must determine if the benefits of the drug outweigh its potentially detrimental aspects. For instance, will the user's detoxification system (liver, kidney, skin, lungs, and gastrointestinal tract) withstand the exposure to the drug, especially if there is long-term use?

The problem occurs when it is time to decide whether to tolerate the anxiety or take a drug and relieve it (assuming the drug works). When you are overwhelmed with anxiety, the risk of dependency and addiction is the furthest thing from your mind. However, that is the danger of drugs, as the need for immediate relief overwhelms concern about future problems.

Untold numbers of patients never go off psychotropic drugs because many of them are afraid they can't do without them. Others who try to discontinue the drugs can't tolerate the discomfort of the transition and often restart them. How-

ever, a large number of doctors are of the opinion that a lifetime of legal drug use may be necessary, arguing that drugs
help avoid anxiety and that outcome is preferable to a lifetime
of suffering. Thus, many patients remain on such medications
indefinitely.

Suppressing symptoms vs. restoring normality. Finally, you
should know that drugs do not restore normal functions to the
brain. Drugs suppress symptoms, but they do *not* restore biochemical and neurological normality. Psychotropic drugs are
not designed to get you to a place where you don't need drugs.
They are designed to suppress your symptoms as long as you
take them—*period.* Quite often, the symptoms return soon
after you discontinue the drug. This is a known fact in medical literature, and this is why many institutions recommend
that you learn and use one or more of the psychological (talk)
techniques mentioned earlier in this chapter. The idea is to
eventually learn how to alter your coping skills to control anxiety without drugs.

I know the majority of the time when a physician writes a
prescription for an anti-anxiety agent he does not automatically refer the patient to a trained therapist for counseling to
develop self-help skills. Perhaps physicians have lost confidence in psychological programs that often fail to work.

Many doctors believe that if a drug suppresses a complaint,
the problem is solved. The new "artificial normal" (calmed
symptoms) created by the drug is sufficient to the patient and
doctor. However, no one is thinking about the fact that the
drug merely postpones the patient's facing a bigger problem
later (addiction, dependency, withdrawal symptoms, anxiety).

WHY MY APPROACH IS DIFFERENT

While some conventionally trained physicians use only pharmaceuticals for treating anxiety, my approach is different and is based on the chemical makeup of anxiety. Through years of research and trial and error, I've found that drugs simply do not provide the body with the extra neurotransmitters needed to block anxiety symptoms. Instead, medications fool the body into temporarily *thinking* it has more neurotransmitters than it really does. The drugs do this by redistributing the neurotransmitters, so that soon after taking the drugs the anxiety symptoms decrease.

Sure, drug therapy works for acute symptoms to calm down a highly anxious person. Moreover, medications are convenient for the physician, as he or she may never have to deal with a patient's anxiety with long-term therapy. Nevertheless, over time, the body can slowly run out of its supply of neurotransmitters, rendering a previously effective drug obsolete. Then where do you go for relief? To understand how this happens, let's look at the three types of neurotransmitters:

1. Simple amino acids that act directly on nerve receptors;
2. Neuropeptides, endorphins, and enkephalins (pain-related agents); and
3. Monoamines, serotonin and dopamine, epinephrine (epi) and norepinephrine (nor-epi).

In general, the neurotransmitters serotonin and dopamine have a calming effect, while epi (also known as adrenaline) and nor-epi (nor-adrenaline) are stimulating. However, in relation to anxiety, aren't we looking for a more calming effect and less stimulation? The answer is yes . . . and no. Serotonin and dopamine are clearly helpful as calming agents, but epi and nor-epi (which are stimulating) are indirectly helpful in another crucial way.

First, epi and nor-epi provide the anxiety patient with mental and physical energy, a necessary factor in overcoming any problem. Secondly, epi and nor-epi are essential for mental clarity. The level of stimulation they provide must be controlled, of course, and epi and nor-epi should not be overly abundant for obvious reasons.

To reduce anxiety, you must balance all four of these neurotransmitters (serotonin, dopamine, epi, and nor-epi). While the neurotransmitters can be affected by drugs, the volume of neurotransmitters present also can be influenced by diet and supplements, two major components of my 5-step holistic program.

Most nerves travel in neuronal bundles of just a few, but the number can go up into the thousands. Try to think of these bundles as electrical cables that are composed of many wires, packed together, just below the outer coating. If there is a loss of power in sufficient numbers of nerves within a bundle, then it will not function efficiently. Epi and nor-epi are energizing neurotransmitters that provide the extra power needed to increase the outflow of messages from the neuronal bundles. When anxiety surfaces, it can feel like every nerve in your body is overly excited. This happens because past assaults on your mental stability from nutritional deficiencies, stress, toxic chemicals, or prolonged drug use have severely taxed your neurotransmitter system and can actually force some of your neuronal bundles off line and they will temporarily cease functioning.

"So, isn't there simply a pill one can take to add the missing neurotransmitters—so that the anxiety will resolve itself?"

If only it worked that way. Neurotransmitters are not available for clinical use, even with a prescription. Still, we can access them another way—that is, from the key nutrients contained in both foods and supplements.

To clarify, the word "nutrient" means a substance that nourishes the body and promotes or sustains life, growth, or strength. A food is any nourishing substance that is eaten, drunk, or otherwise taken into the body to provide energy and sustenance. Likewise, natural dietary supplements contain one or more dietary ingredients (including vitamins; minerals; herbs or other botanicals; amino acids; and other substances) or their constituents.

For the most part, using foods to boost neurotransmitters is out because none has the concentrations of amino acids and cofactors (described below) we are looking for. Sure, meats have plenty of amino acids, but they're not balanced toward any specific neurotransmitter, so they end up only serving as an energy source.

Nevertheless, therapists have long employed supplemental amino acids as foundation materials for the formation of various neurotransmitters. A precursor is a nutrient that acts as raw material for use by the body in making a neurotransmitter. To be effective, each precursor nutrient requires the necessary cofactors: vitamins, minerals, and other nutrients. A cofactor is a material that must accompany the precursor in order for the precursor to work. For instance, the precursor to serotonin is the nutrient 5-hydroxytryptophan or 5-HTP, which must be accompanied by the cofactor vitamin B_6 or the nutrient cannot be converted into serotonin. Vitamin B_6 works as a cofactor in more than 100 enzyme reactions, particularly those related to the metabolism of amino acids and other proteins. This B vitamin affects the synthesis of serotonin and dopamine, neurotransmitters necessary for healthy nerve cell communication. (To learn more about how nutrients work, consult Step 2, in Chapter 6.)

Understanding Terms

· *Nutrient*—A substance that nourishes the body and promotes or sustains life, growth, or strength.
· *Food*—Any nourishing substance that is eaten, drunk, or otherwise taken into the body to provide energy and sustenance.
· *Natural dietary supplement*—A substance that contains one or more dietary ingredients (including vitamins; minerals; herbs or other botanicals; amino acids; and other substances) or their constituents.

Balance Your Brain's Chemistry Naturally

Over the past three decades, I have learned that by working to balance the above-mentioned neurotransmitters, it's possible to decrease or eliminate nearly every form of anxiety naturally. Of course, no treatment is guaranteed, and everyone responds differently; but overall, the process is successful in a large number of cases. My approach to neurotransmitter therapy should always be used in conjunction with the additional support remedies mentioned in my 5-step program such as getting quality sleep, exercising daily, eating a proper diet, and using essential fatty acids.

Before I discuss neurotransmitters let me clarify a possible area of confusion. Isolated numbers and letters can sometimes become confusing so let me elaborate on two similar symbols: 5-HTP (note the "P") is the symbol for the chemical 5-hydroxy tryptophane, an amino acid found in food and used in nutritional supplements; 5-HT (note the absence of the "P") is the symbol for 5-hydroxy tryptamine or serotonin (a brain neurotransmitter). So there you have it, 5-HTP (amino acid) is ingested in food and is then converted in the brain to 5-HT (serotonin).

Now let's review how nutrients can influence neurotransmitters:

Serotonin. Anytime anxiety is a problem the first neurotransmitter that comes to mind is serotonin. Serotonin (5-HT) supervises all of the other neurotransmitters, so obviously it is one of the more important workers in our body's chemistry, especially the chemistry related to feelings. When you have optimal levels of serotonin, you are in a good mood and not stressed by worry.

But when you have too little serotonin, it is a different story. Anxiety, depression, obsessive-compulsiveness, and insomnia are only a few of the symptoms that occur when you are deficient. I need to make two simple but important points here:

1. Low serotonin is one part of an anxiety problem; and
2. The body can produce serotonin easily once you supply it with the right precursor materials (i.e., nutrients).

Knowing this, it makes fixing this part of the problem relatively simple. I say "this part," because a serotonin deficiency is often only a *partial* cause for anxiety. The rule of thumb in this type of therapy is that all four of the important neurotransmitters (serotonin, dopamine, epi, and nor-epi) need to be in balance for any one of them to exert its optimal effect.

Years ago the amino acid tryptophan was readily available as a supplement at most natural food stores. I used tryptophan exclusively to raise serotonin levels, asking patients to take 500 to 1,000 milligrams of tryptophan and at the same time to eat something sugary or sweet. Upon doing this, we just had to wait a little while for the brain to produce its own serotonin.

Today, tryptophan is no longer available without a prescription, so another natural dietary supplement called 5-hydroxytryptophan or 5-HTP (pages 160–161) is a safe substitute. This over-the-counter supplement is found in most natural food stores and, when taken, the 5-HTP goes straight into the brain, making itself immediately available to be converted into serotonin.

When you ingest 5-HTP with the intention of increasing serotonin, in a sense you are taking an antidepressant remedy. Most of the major antidepressant medications work by increasing serotonin (and other neurotransmitters, too). While 5-HTP does not have nearly the potency of a drug, it clearly does have proven effects—without the potentially dangerous side effects of drugs. That is why I use 5-HTP in my practice instead of drugs to treat anxiety patients with a serotonin deficiency, including those with anxiety, depression, and sleep problems.

Antidepressants and anti-anxiety nutrients usually take between two days and two weeks to be effective. Similarly, 5-HTP may work immediately, the next day, or it may not work for two months; each person is different. Anti-anxiety drugs, on average, have a faster onset. However, drugs, being concentrated chemicals, are prone to side effects; 5-HTP and other similar natural dietary supplements seldom cause any problems. Because vitamin B_6 is the cofactor of 5-HTP, you must take at last 50 milligrams a day for the 5-HTP to convert into serotonin. Remember: Neurotransmitters work in teams.

Dopamine, epinephrine, and nor-epinephrine. Dopamine, another key neurotransmitter, promotes a sense of well-being. When we have enough dopamine, we feel great. When we have too little dopamine, we develop symptoms of depression and anxiety.

Our body uses the nutrients we eat to manufacture millions of molecules of dopamine every day. Most of the time when we lack the right nutrient to make dopamine, it's because our body is using more of the essential material than normal; our needs outpace our supply. In other words, utilization exceeds what a normal diet can offer.

One example of over-utilization is the depletion of brain chemicals in the process of metabolizing drugs. The body requires considerable amounts of nutrients to move drugs through and finally out of our system. It doesn't matter whether the drugs are prescription or recreational. Either way, drug processing may be using up more brain nutrients than normal, and so we end up chronically deficient. Stress can do the same thing. The bottom line is you may find yourself fresh out of building materials just when you need them most.

In the biochemistry of neurotransmitters it turns out that dopamine is the precursor to epi and nor-epi. Therefore, it stands to reason that anything that increases dopamine automatically also increases epi and nor-epi. The precursor to dopamine is a combination of the two amino acids tyrosine and phenylalanine. These two amino acids are thought to create significant mood change, since dopamine, which is generated from these precursors, is involved in anxiety and depression. Other amino acids such as L-lysine and L-arginine are thought to alleviate stress anxiety.

The cofactor for tyrosine and phenylalanine is the B complex vitamins. You will soon notice in Step 2 (Chapter 6) of my program, that I frequently utilize B vitamins to reduce anxiety, as they help improve neurotransmitter balance.

The point to all this is that I have found that properly selected nutrients can make a difference in the level of brain chemicals available for use. If your body gets what it needs, then it can make what it needs in the brain as easily as it does in the rest of the body. Some people are born with a greater need than others, and they are what we call nutrient-dependent. They will always need to ingest more of the precursors to the essential brain chemical than the rest of us.

Importance of Precursor Nutrients

As you follow my natural approach to treating anxiety, you will learn that to rebalance the body, you must decide which precursor nutrients would be useful. If you misjudge and eat the wrong foods or take the wrong supplement, you can make things worse. That's why it's vital to talk with your doctor or a qualified expert to make sure the nutrients are right for your situation.

MULTIFACETED NATURAL APPROACH

As you start my program, you will see how each step builds upon the others, giving you a complete roadmap to easing anxiety and strengthening the body. Because the program is a multifaceted natural approach, as opposed to a one-dimensional drug approach, it offers many therapies—sometimes even very simple answers—that can help ease anxiety and related symptoms.

For example, recently a young woman named Maki came to me complaining of chronic anxiety and depression. During the workup, I asked her if there were any foods she craved. I had learned from long experience that the foods you crave might be the very foods to which you are allergic-sensitive. By eating them, you're suppressing withdrawal symptoms and thus avoiding an acute reaction. Maki said she loved tuna, especially in sushi. She ate it numerous times a day and it lifted her spirits.

As a home test, I asked Maki not to eat any tuna for four days and then on the fifth day to resume regular consumption (see full description of the neurotoxicity test on p. 116). Two weeks later, she came to the clinic and explained the results of this clinical or home trial. During the four days of withdrawal from tuna, she became fatigued. Then she slowly felt a growing relief from her anxiety and depression. On the fifth day, Maki had her first bowl of tuna and she deliberately made it a large portion. Within a half-hour, she was morbidly depressed. She then experienced a wave of anxiety and began to sob. She cried throughout the day and into the night and finally, exhausted, fell asleep in the early morning. She woke up feeling better and did not resume the tuna after that. Now, after a week without tuna, her anxiety and depression were greatly reduced.

If every case were this clear-cut, my book would only be about the treatment of food and chemical sensitivities! Let's look at the case of twenty-one-year-old Liz, who came to my clinic with complaints of chronic depression and anxiety. This young college student wasn't suicidal, but she could never seem to find anything to be happy about. She was raised in a relatively normal, stress-free family and had a promising future. Liz said that she slept well, and there was nothing of note in her medical history.

When I ran some laboratory tests, I found that Liz's testosterone (male hormone) level was low. I put this young woman on a low dose of testosterone. When I saw her seven days later, she said that two days after she started the testosterone she began to feel better. Now, just one week later, she was completely free of her anxiety and depression.

Granted, most of the cases I see are much more complex than Maki's and Liz's. Nonetheless, I share these to make a strong point. Had these young women visited a traditional doctor, they would have possibly received the same anti-anxiety/antidepressant medication. Instead, the women wanted to understand their own bodies. They learned to evaluate their lifestyle and diet habits, and then consider various solutions in order to find the right one that was natural and long-term without deleterious side effects.

Nutritional Supplements Are a Large Component

Dietary supplements used in my multifaceted program are concentrates of specific elements found within foods. Herbs, for example, can be used as spices in cooking or as a remedy for a health problem. The herb ginger adds zest to cookies, pies, and various dishes and has a calming influence on the stomach when used to quell nausea. While we take most vitamins for granted in the foods we eat, if you are lacking vitamin B_{12}, you might suffer with memory loss, confusion, listlessness, and even hallucinations. Vitamin B_{12} is vital for health and the life of every cell and bodily system. Moreover, vitamin B_{12} increases energy and can help prevent depression in the elderly.

A nutritional supplement can be made from dozens of different classes of natural materials, including vitamins, minerals, amino acids, proteins, fats or fatty acids, bee by-products, lichens, herbs, kelp and other ocean plants, salt and other mineral deposits, and shell by-products, among others. But while whole foods can be useful in reducing anxiety, I find that supplements are much easier to deal with compared to preparing, transporting, or preserving foods. Therefore, while I will mention whole foods in my multifaceted program, the emphasis will be on natural supplements.

A Note About Safety

Anything that nourishes the body is safe in proportion. For instance, the proper amount of the mineral zinc nourishes the body. However, a large amount can be poisonous. This risk occurs only when the material is misused. There is no risk from nutrients when used properly. This is in stark contrast to a drug, which can carry a risk even when used correctly. Fortunately, the proper amount of each nutrient is well documented, so we are easily able to limit our intake to the levels that only provide nourishment. I will elaborate on this later.

A Combination Approach

As I said earlier, I do use drugs in some cases, especially when I have an especially discouraged person with marginal commitment to a nondrug approach (noncompliance). I prescribe drugs for short periods until the nutritional approach kicks in. I use drugs intermittently with nutritional approaches to manage flare-ups between periods of stability when the level of anxiety exhibited requires an acutely effective remedy.

Occasionally I will mix drugs and nutrients for optimal results. For instance, I recently treated a woman who was unable to sleep without taking Xanax (alprazolam) combined with another tranquilizer that her family doctor prescribed. I respected the other doctor's work and did not attempt to change this prescription; rather, I gave it a little boost. When I added a nutrient to the woman's nightly routine, her sleep became completely normalized and enriching. In this case, I used a nutrient to boost the drug effect. However, the majority of the time I don't need to use drugs while treating an anxiety disorder.

Should you choose to use a nutritional approach instead of or in addition to drug therapy, be sure to inform all your doctors. Give each doctor a list of all natural dietary supplements and drugs you take to make sure you don't have a drug-nutrient interaction.

When Drugs Are Needed Along with the Nutritional Approach

- Drugs are needed in cases where the anxiety is associated with another major mental disturbance such as bipolar disorder, schizophrenia, or psychotic depression.
- Drugs should be used in any situation where an attending physician believes it is necessary and essential to the control of a serious anxiety.
- Drugs should be used in any case where there is a danger to the person in question or to others.

- Drugs are required when all nutritional approaches have failed.
- Drugs are the solution when there has been non-compliance with the nutritional approach, meaning the patient cannot stay with the plan.

Nutrient Potency

Most drugs originate from native plants from various regions, the Amazon jungle being the most famous. Plants, from which most nutrients are derived, manufacture mind-altering chemicals for self-protection; an insect or an animal that feels strange after eating a plant will not eat that plant again—the plant has defended itself against another attack.

You might question whether available nutrients are strong enough in their present form to do any good. The answer? They certainly are. One very good example is the amino acid tryptophan (page 88). Most experts report that 500 to 1,000 milligrams of tryptophan will have a strong sedating effect on virtually anyone. When taken properly, this amino acid is a superb sleep aid.

The Potency of Natural Dietary Supplements

- Nutrients cannot be exchanged one for one with a drug, but they may have a high degree of potency.
- Since nutrients are less potent than drugs, gram for gram, a nutrient must be taken in larger amounts for a discernible effect.
- In addition to providing relief from symptoms, nutrient

benefits are derived from positive molecular changes (those that take place in the smallest physical units of our tissues).
- Nutrient benefits result in overall health upgrades, which protect us against all illnesses.
- The nutrient approach is most effective if our goal is to arrive at a new balance in our body's chemistry.

Definition of a Natural Dietary Supplement

According to the Food and Drug Administration, in order for an ingredient of a dietary supplement to be what's referred to as a dietary ingredient, it must be one or any combination of the following substances:

- vitamin
- mineral
- herb or other botanical
- amino acid
- dietary substance for use by man to supplement diet by increasing the total dietary intake (i.e., enzymes or tissues from organs or glands)
- concentrate, metabolite, constituent, or extract

Lasting Treatment Without Adverse Effects

Please note that my 5-step program will not stop symptoms as fast as Xanax or other pharmaceuticals. I've only seen a few occasions when nutrients offered immediate anxiety relief. Yet the natural therapies can be tremendously valuable over time by helping to restore much of the body's normal homeostatic balance (internal stability) and natural control over emotions—without adverse effects. I believe that when the body is strengthened, so is the emotional state, and this is the ultimate goal of my program.

For many, a short-term situational anxiety can easily and efficiently be controlled with a prescription medication. But most of my patients have permanent generalized anxiety with other disorders such as agoraphobia and panic attacks. Many patients come to me with one or more prescriptions from their family doctor. And no matter how well the drugs work, the patients still feel trapped in a body that is frequently out of control.

Again, while patients do benefit from drugs, often the results are not enough to give excellent quality of life. When patients come to my office, they talk about wanting freedom from disease, not a life where drugs stand between them and their misery. In addition, side effects are extremely common, as discussed on pages 11–14.

HOW TO USE MY 5-STEP HOLISTIC PROGRAM

Now that you have a good idea of why I believe in a natural, multidimensional approach to resolving anxiety, go ahead and turn to my holistic program in Part 2 of this book. I do not suggest that you attempt to utilize all the information in this book, but rather only the parts that apply to you. The reason there are so many areas to consider is that a plethora of approaches provides us with a rich warehouse of natural therapies from which to choose.

In my clinic, I make the prescriptive choices for the patient; here, in this book, I can only guide you so far. Every therapy mentioned in this book has alleviated anxiety in many of my patients. However, ultimately, you must work with your doctors to choose the most appropriate approach that applies in your situation. I strongly suggest that you also talk with your doctor before taking any natural dietary supplement, and insist that you never stop prescribed medication without discussing doing so first with your doctor.

There's no one answer to relieving anxiety disorders. My program focuses on many natural therapies and lifestyle changes that only you can make. However, the ultimate reward of living a life without anxiety, phobias, and panic—and without the adverse effects of strong pharmaceuticals—will be well worth most any sacrifice.

In the chapters to follow, we will form a team committed to relieving your individual symptoms and improving your quality of life. Now let's get to work!

Part 2

DR. HUNT'S 5-STEP
HOLISTIC PROGRAM

Chapter 5

〰️

Step 1: Get an Accurate Diagnosis

When Kim finally came to my clinic, she had suffered with crippling anxiety and panic for more than two years. At thirty-three-years old, she had recently taken a leave of absence from her job as an accountant and moved back home with her parents because of increasingly debilitating fears.

After listening to Kim's symptoms of ongoing anxiety, disrupted sleep, and daily panic attacks, ruling out other serious problems with a few laboratory tests, I diagnosed Kim with generalized anxiety disorder (GAD) and panic attacks without agorophobia. I immediately started her on my B complex injections and had her use the Body Control peppermint spray (four to six mouth sprays) if she felt anxiety or panicky (see Resources). She also took 300 mg of magnesium three times a day and 50 mg of 5-hydroxytryptophan (5-HTP), (pages 160–161), a dietary supplement that has a calming effect, three times a day. Once Kim was stabilized, she began to use other effective natural remedies explained in my program. Even though she realized that there would be no instant end to the symptoms until her body's biochemistry was in balance again, Kim was relieved that she was finally gaining control over a problem that stole her productivity and active young life.

As with any medical condition, an accurate diagnosis must always precede treatment. In the case of anxiety disorders, there are three levels of diagnosis required before beginning treatment.

1. *First level:* Classify the existing disease according to the traditional medical model;
2. *Second level:* Uncover the primary weakness or a group of weaknesses in the body and mind that exaggerate and perpetuate the anxiety disorders; and
3. *Third level:* Set up a short- and long-term treatment plan. The short-term goal is to take appropriate and immediate anxiety-relieving steps; the long-term goal is to rehabilitate a dysfunctional nervous system.

YOUR PERSONAL MENTAL HEALTH CONSULTATION

As you seek an accurate diagnosis of the cause and type of anxiety disorder, select a doctor whom you can trust to take responsibility for your overall mental health. This may be a conventional medical doctor or an alternative medicine specialist. Be sure you can talk openly with this man or woman about your symptoms and concerns.

In my clinic, I begin the quest of an accurate diagnosis by talking with the patient. This lengthy process requires a detailed personal medical history, including information on anxiety and related symptoms, medical history and medications, exercise and activity level, diet and eating habits, home and work environment, and the patient's family medical history.

Because some forms of anxiety disorder such as panic attacks and social phobia have a genetic tendency, it is important to know if parents, siblings, or other close relatives also have similar signs and symptoms.

With today's high-tech medicine, we are used to special tests to arrive at a diagnosis. However, most laboratory tests are not very helpful by themselves in making the diagnosis of anxiety disorders. In fact, diagnosing anxiety disorders is completely different from detecting a medical problem. For example, if you have a sore throat, the doctor can culture a throat swab to determine which bacteria are causing the infection. Once the exact germ is known, a specific medication can be given that is known to eradicate that bacteria. With anxiety disorders, there is no specific battery of diagnostic tests or medications known to stop symptoms every time. While we have laboratory tests and scans that might prove useful in accurately assessing the patient's mental and physical health, for the most part we must rely on a combination of discussion, tests, if needed, and trial and error of various medications or natural therapies to find what works to resolve the problem.

The following section will give you an idea of the customary procedure used to evaluate anxiety disorders. You can share this information with your conventional medical doctor or alternative care specialist to help get an accurate diagnosis.

Signs and Symptoms

The specialist you choose will seek an accurate diagnosis by obtaining a detailed personal medical history, including an inventory of your anxiety symptoms. During this evaluation, it's important that you are up-front about the feelings of anxiety, fear, panic, phobias, or worries, and how the anxiety disorder manifests itself in your case. This will allow your doctor to have a firm understanding of your anxiety problem and will be the basis for the treatment plan. Some questions your doctor might ask include the following:

1. When did you first experience your symptom or symptoms?
2. Can you describe what you feel (nervous, paranoid, overwhelmed, pounding heart, difficulty breathing, facial flushing)?
3. Do you know what caused the symptom to develop?
4. How long did the symptom or symptoms last?
5. Was there anything at the time that relieved the symptoms?
6. From the first attack to now, how many times has it returned? How long does it last each time?
7. Do you experience the symptom hourly, daily, weekly, or monthly?
8. Do you have a family history of anxiety disorders?
9. What are you taking or doing for it now?
10. To what degree is the symptom interfering with your personal, social, or occupational life today?

Sleep Hygiene

Because insomnia and sleep disorders are almost universal in anxiety and panic patients, sleep hygiene should be considered. Many times anxiety sufferers' sleep is dysfunctional in that they cannot get to sleep or they awaken frequently throughout the night. The good news is that with the appropriate natural therapy, most patients finally get healing sleep, and anxiety and related symptoms often improve up to 50 percent.

Medical History and Medications

Medical conditions such as underactive thyroid, hypoglycemia, or anemia and medications used to treat many illnesses can also explain anxiety symptoms. Your doctor will inquire about your medical and medication history during the evaluation:

1. What, if any, drug or nutrients are you taking now?
2. How does each benefit you or bother you?
3. Have you been exposed to a toxic chemical or aerosol recently or in the past?
4. Do you have a chronic disease related to fungus (mold) or a virus?
5. Have you ever suffered extreme exhaustion from mental stress, trauma, pregnancy, or illness?
6. Is your family susceptible to the same symptoms you suffer now?
7. Are you bothered by pollen, chemical, or food sensitivities?
8. Have you had any hormonal problems related to birth control pills, menopause, menstrual irregularities, and so on?

Drugs and Alcohol

It's important for your doctor to know if you have a history of alcohol or drug misuse. Ingesting excessive caffeine, herbal stimulants, recreational drugs, prescription drugs, and alcohol could all be the source of anxiety. The good news is that eliminating this source might easily resolve your anxiety problem.

Other Factors to Consider

Whether you see a conventional medical doctor or an alternative care specialist, the principle of diagnosis preceding treatment is observed. While the conventional doctor might rely on medications and talk therapy for healing, the alternative care physician will apply the more natural approaches, as described in my program, to ensure optimal health and healing. Here are other lifestyle and health factors that your doctor might consider during the patient consultation:

Energy. Your doctor might ask you about your energy level for a good reason: You can't make appropriate judgments when your mind is weak from lack of energy. In fact, the lower your physical and mental strength, the more difficult it is to manage emotions.

Allergies and chemical sensitivities. It's important to know if you have any allergies or chemical sensitivities. I have found that nutritional support (described in my program) enhances the immune and the detoxification systems. When you experience optimal health, the level of your anxiety will be reduced.

Diet. Talk openly with your doctor about your diet, including any natural dietary supplements you take. A diet high in simple carbohydrates (simple sugar) can cause fluctuations in blood sugar levels, resulting in mood swings and physical weakness. Drinking too much caffeine can greatly increase anxiety in susceptible people. And sometimes a poor diet can result in low energy or difficulty maintaining sleep. All of this influences your emotional stamina. A detailed set of nutritional guidelines can be found in Chapter 7.

Musculoskeletal involvement. Discuss the level of musculoskeletal involvement in your anxiety. Are the muscles a dominant factor? Is the anxiety more cerebral? Fibromyalgia (an arthritis-like syndrome), chronic fatigue, and autoimmune diseases such as lupus or rheumatoid arthritis are frequently accompanied by anxiety. As with all anxiety-related diseases, your doctor needs to look for any underlying disease and address this as well as the anxiety.

Gastrointestinal candida infection. Any chronic or long-term infection weakens the immune system and that impacts anxiety levels. Although I've had just a few patients where the elimination of candida reversed the symptoms of anxiety or panic, this condition is one your doctor might want to rule out.

Narrowing the Diagnosis

No matter what symptoms you have, your doctor will act like a medical detective, trying to solve the anxiety mystery. As you give information about your medical history and emotional experiences, your doctor will narrow the anxiety disorder into a specific diagnosis, such as panic disorder, phobias, or adjustment disorder, among others. Most of the time, a diagnosis is relatively simple and can even be aided by your awareness of mental health issues. It's highly common for patients to look up their diagnosis on Internet mental health sites and develop a fairly sophisticated knowledge of the problem before they even see a health care professional.

Using the answers in the previous section, you can assist your doctor in narrowing down your diagnosis. I give a few examples of specific anxiety disorders below. For more detailed information on the most common disorders, read Chapters 2 and 3.

Panic attack. If you have panic attacks along with a great deal of worry, your doctor might consider whether the panic is in conjunction with agoraphobia. For example, if you stay at home to avoid a panic attack, agoraphobia is a likely diagnosis. If you are not housebound, then the diagnosis might be panic disorder without agoraphobia. Your doctor may try to determine if your panic symptoms are clustered around social situations or performance obligations. If so, you might have a social phobia disorder with the panic.

Phobias. Most people are aware of specific phobias and social phobias, so in the case of a phobic patient, the diagnosis is usually quick and to the point. If you avoid a specific situation or social encounter, your doctor might consider that you have a specific phobia.

Obsessions and compulsions. Most people who come to see me are well informed about obsessive-compulsive disorder and either suspect or know they have this problem. Before you decide that you are OCD, it's important that someone with clinical training review your symptoms and make an accurate diagnosis. The problem is that there are no laboratory tests for OCD. I use some written tests for those suspected of having this disorder, but these tests just confirm what is already apparent. Laboratory tests such as exposure to carbon dioxide or sodium lactate to determine serum levels are only performed in a research setting and are not available to the practicing physician.

Generalized anxiety disorder. If your symptoms of worry, fear, and heightened arousal have been steady for six months or more and are not focused on a specific cause, then you probably have a generalized anxiety disorder (GAD). In my practice, when I get to this point in the consultation, I want to make sure that the patient's problem isn't more serious. Because the closest relative to an anxiety disorder is a mood disorder, I inquire about episodes of depression or elevated moods alternating with depression (bipolar disorder) and symptoms related to a smaller group such as schizoaffective disorder, cyclothymic disorder, and dysthymic disorder. With schizoaffective disorder, a cross between schizophrenia and bipolar disease, the patient's symptoms range between depression, mania, and the psychotic symptoms of schizophrenia. One phase may dominate at any time but the other symptoms are always underlying them. Cyclothymic disorder is characterized by at least two years of minimum to moderate manic symptoms interspersed between numerous periods of mild to moderate depression. Dysthymic disorder causes symptoms such as years of mild to moderate depression that occurs more days than not.

Stress disorders. It's important that your doctor rule out the possibility of a major depression or a psychosis. I ask about the possibility of a single or a series of traumatic events that have changed the way the patient views the world. Such an event could cause acute stress disorder, adjustment disorder, or post-traumatic stress disorder, all discussed in Chapter 3.

During the initial patient consultation, I can usually determine early on whether I am the right person to help the patient or if he or she should be referred to another health care professional. For instance, if the patient has anxiety but is also schizophrenic, bipolar, or psychotically depressed, I refer the patient to a mental health clinic in my area that specializes in these more serious pathologies. If the anxiety problem appears to be organic (neurological), then I refer the patient to a neurologist.

If you have been diagnosed with or suffer with any of the following behaviors, then this book is *not* for you: psychosis, schizophrenia, psychotic depression, borderline personality, bipolar disorder, substance abuse disorder, or attention deficit disorder (ADD). Talk with your doctor about appropriate therapy.

DR. HUNT'S HOLISTIC RX: GETTING AN ACCURATE DIAGNOSIS

In my clinic, after a thorough discussion with the patient, I use one or more of the following assessments with anxiety patients, depending on signs and symptoms and medical history:

- Complete blood panel
- Hormone levels
- Health status blood testing (for thyroid problems)
- Glucose tolerance test (for diabetes and hypoglycemia)
- Albumin/Globulin (for immune dysfunction)
- Kidney and liver function tests (for overall patient health)
- Cholesterol and triglyceride screening (low cholesterol is associated with depression)
- EEG, CT, MRI, and SPECT scans (described below)
- Sleep study (polysomnography)
- Vitamin and mineral levels
- Neurotransmitter analysis
- Fatty acid analysis
- Digestive and stool profile
- Toxic metal test

In the following sections, I will discuss these and other tests and how they might help your doctor make an accurate diagnosis. After reviewing these tests, talk openly with your doctor about specific assessments you might need. Once a diagnosis has been made, consider the treatment modalities given in Steps 2 to 5 to regain your health, energy, and productive life.

ANXIETY AND TESTING

Depending on your symptoms and discussion, your doctor might choose to order laboratory tests. Sometimes the tests are ordered so your doctor can exclude more serious medical problems.

The only standard lab tests that I order routinely are the complete blood panel and a test for gender hormones. The complete blood panel, a standard laboratory test, measures the hemoglobin, red cells, white cells, and platelets and can also find many of the common blood disorders, which can cause fatigue and tiredness.

With a complete blood panel, I look for anemia, thyroid problems, bacterial, viral, or fungal infections, immune resistance, liver and kidney dysfunctions, cholesterol status, diabetes or hypoglycemia, malnutrition, and weak adrenal strength, among other problems. The gender hormone test checks the levels of estrogen, progesterone, free testosterone, DHEA (dehydroepiandrosterone), and DHEAS (dehydroepiandrosterone sulfate).

Unless there is an organic (physical) reason behind the anxiety, your doctor might evaluate your ability to detoxify the drug of choice and only order further testing if there were some reason to suspect liver, kidney, or other organ involvement.

Imaging Tests

Using the results of your medical history and routine blood tests, your doctor may order more tests to eliminate a more serious problem like cancer. The following high-tech imaging tests are often used:

• **Electroencephalogram (EEG)**—With the EEG, electrodes are placed on the scalp over different areas of the brain to record patterns of electrical activity. This graphic record can detect abnormal brain wave activity and is used to eliminate the presence of a growth (tumor), infection, seizure disorder, or metabolic disorder as a cause for anxiety. The EEG can also indicate the presence of dementia or Alzheimer's disease, which often shows slower than normal brain waves. It is also used when areas of abnormal electrical activity in the brain occur such as with diseases like encephalitis.

• **Computerized axial tomography (CAT scan)**—The CAT scan consists of a series of X-rays taken from many angles as the machine circles the head of the patient. After hundreds of X-rays are taken, they are analyzed by a computer to generate a three-dimensional picture many times more detailed than a typical X-ray. The picture is able to clearly expose, with pinpoint accuracy, any area of the brain or any object that is of interest. This neuroimaging test examines the structure of the brain and may be ordered to eliminate a physical cause for anxiety, such as evidence of strokes, blood clots in the brain, tumors, or head injuries. The CAT scan is used for sinusitis, especially when accompanied by dizziness, weakness, or a strange feeling in the head, and for constant headaches, especially when they occur with anxiety.

• **Magnetic resonance imaging (MRI) scans**—With an MRI, radioactive material (less than contained in a single

X-ray) is injected in the vein of the patient. Then a strong magnetic field is passed through the brain while pictures are being taken. The scanner in the machine can detect radiation from certain molecules in organs that remove them from the blood and concentrate them. Extremely reliable, the pictures taken will conclusively eliminate the possibility of tumors or other physical disturbances in the brain as a cause of anxiety. The MRI is also used to assess activity or lack thereof in areas of the brain such as the basal ganglia, which relate to anxiety.

• **X-rays**—X-rays were used in the past as another way to eliminate physical causes for anxiety but they have mostly been replaced by the tests just mentioned.

• **Ultrasound**—Ultrasound images are used frequently on glands such as the thyroid to eliminate physical causes of anxiety. A thyroid tumor, for example, might produce overactivity, which would result in anxiety.

Psychological Testing

There are many psychological tests that determine the levels of anxiety and depression, but these tests are seldom used. After all, you know if you are anxious or not and how bad it is. In most cases, the therapist depends more on a continuing relationship with the patient for a clearer picture of the problem.

Psychological testing is probably most useful in determining personality characteristics, since these factors play a large role in adaptability, motivation for change, secondary gain, and any other character trait that might weaken, undermine, or even strengthen successful mental illness therapy.

There is a different type of mental abilities testing that is frequently performed in the educational system where cerebral and emotional strengths and weaknesses are illuminated. Some educators have indicated, and I agree with them, that when you clearly understand your strengths and weaknesses, you are better prepared to make accurate life decisions and elevate confidence while lowering anxiety. Most people would have less anxiety if they were living a life closer to their native abilities, thus reducing unnecessary conflicts. For a person to function optimally in their personal, family, social, or occupational life they must be able to take information in, retain it, and then properly express the information. There are a number of mental tasks that make this process proceed smoothly.

If your doctor feels that psychological testing is necessary, you should consider it. An under-functioning area of the brain, not detectable by any of the laboratory tests mentioned above, might be another unrecognized source of anxiety.

ALTERNATIVE CARE TESTING

Alternative care therapists may use any or all of the standard approaches just mentioned, along with other specialized tests when they are applicable. For example, after ordering the blood and hormone tests, discussed on page 111, I may order a sleep study (polysomnography) for patients who suffer with insomnia or other sleep disorders. The sleep study can detect fragmented or broken sleep patterns and determine if the patient is proceeding through the four stages of sleep for an adequate amount of time. It can also find out if shallow breathing is causing under-oxygenation of the blood, resulting in chronic fatigue.

Whenever additional testing is necessary, I ask myself these questions:

1. Will the test results allow me to better help the patient control anxiety?
2. Will the test results significantly contribute to the rehabilitation of the underlying disease?
3. Are the tests worth the money and time?

Before you and your doctor decide to run more tests, you should discuss the three issues above. Most people do not understand that tests are not always completely accurate. The test results are only an approximate level of something that quickly changes over time. In addition, it is difficult to test for anxiety and related problems.

Since we cannot pinpoint exact problems with test results, then, at best, these results are only moderately helpful. Therefore, the question remains, is the test worth doing at all? With this thought in mind, I will explain some of the tests alternative doctors utilize. I should mention that there are hundreds of tests, so I can only present a representative few.

Nutrition Panel

A nutrition panel is a test commonly used by alternative medicine practitioners. This test examines vitamin and mineral levels, fatty acids, amino acids, organic acids, gastrointestinal functions, oxidant stress levels, and detoxification capacity. This test is pricey, as you might expect. However, if it gives you the shortcut to relieving anxiety, I'm sure you would think the price was worth it! Still, it is not always this easy. While you might feel better taking the supplements indicated by the panel, your anxiety would be only slightly affected, and the long-term benefits would only be partial.

First, there is nothing in conventional or alternative medicine journals that indicates simply achieving higher levels of health automatically removes anxiety. Many healthy people suffer anxiety. Practical experience substantiates this concept. Aiming strictly for superior health fails to correct mental problems, including anxiety. It is the extremes outside your normal healthy chemistry that we must address and, although correcting generalized nutritional imbalances strengthens mental health, anxiety is a disease state that completely resists simple remedies like this.

In my experience, each person requires specific nutritional remedies that fall outside general nutritional testing. Not that such testing is bad; it is simply not enough and even may be a distraction from the more productive approaches.

Neurotoxicity Challenge Test

The neurotoxicity challenge test is a home clinical test. With a clinical test, you are asked to perform a task and then record the outcome. Food sensitivity testing is a perfect example of a clinical test.

If you suspect you are reacting adversely to a food, then follow these instructions: Withdraw from the offending food for four days. Abstinence from the suspected food must be absolute. On the fifth day, consume the food in large amounts. For example, if you suspect that milk is an offending food, then you must completely avoid all dairy products such as cheese, yogurt, sour cream, cottage cheese, ice cream, coffee creamer, or any other food that contains milk in even the smallest amounts.

The accuracy of this test depends on you having perfect control of what you eat—and don't eat—during the period of testing. If you do not react on the fifth day when you are overindulging in the suspect food, then chances are you are not sensitive to that food and it can be consumed freely in the future.

Be suspicious of your favorite foods or foods you crave such as sugars, dairy products, grains, including rice and soy, or any other food that you notice experiencing mental or physical changes following its consumption. I recommend to patients that they compile a list and test the foods one at a time rather than all at once.

Perhaps the best way to test for chemical neurotoxicity is to keep a journal of each reaction that happens during your daily life. If a friend's aftershave lotion bothers you, then write down exactly how you felt and how long the symptoms lasted. Now, I'm not referring to symptoms of sneezing or an itchy nose. We are not interested in upper respiratory symptoms but rather symptoms that have to do with mental or emotional changes. Some individuals suffer a rush of irritation from chemical exposure while others respond with a sense of sadness or helplessness. A passing exposure is seldom enough to set off a severe reaction but more than enough to trigger some kind of response. Typical triggering agents include the following:

- cigarette smoke
- cleaning solutions
- gasoline
- newspaper ink
- fabric dyes
- mold
- smog

In my clinic, I do not think it is useful to order food allergy tests or chemical sensitivity tests although there are many physicians who would disagree with me. I believe the home clinical testing described above is more than adequate for most patients.

Neurotransmitter Testing

In testing for neurotransmitters (chemical messengers in the brain), your doctor will use a urine specimen instead of drawing your blood. During a stressful situation, the kidneys allow a large outflowing of neurotransmitters much to the detriment of the brain and body. Given the test results, you can add or subtract nutrients that will increase or decrease the amount of neurotransmitters available to the body based on how much the kidneys excrete.

While no one yet has explained why the kidneys permit this type of loss, we do know that by adding the supporting nutrients that fortify and strengthen the major neurotransmitters, it appears this urinary drain stops. (Normal ranges and optimal ranges have been established on urine specimens.)

This type of laboratory testing is useful because it establishes an ongoing relationship between the test findings and the symptom reports from the patient. Neurotransmitter therapy with therapeutic ranges via precursor supplementation is safer than drug therapy and sometimes faster. It allows many patients to reduce or discontinue drugs altogether. For those who need to stay on drugs, it makes the drugs more effective and prevents the typical loss of effectiveness that usually occurs over time. Lastly, neurotransmitter testing allows many patients to discontinue the nutrient support or substantially reduce the quantity of nutrients they are prescribed.

Neurotransmitter therapy is not a panacea. It can help your doctor determine the excess or deficit of neurotransmitters related to anxiety such as serotonin and dopamine. Once your doctor has the test results, this is used as a baseline for treatment. When it works well, it is wondrous; but it doesn't work on everyone. For this very reason, my 5-step program is multifaceted and focuses on many natural therapies and lifestyle changes rather than on one answer to relieving anxiety disorders.

Gastrointestinal Testing

Gastrointestinal testing is not mandatory in the diagnosis and treatment of an anxiety disorder, yet I believe there are times when it has benefits. This test can determine chronic unrecognized infections such as candida (yeast) or parasites, as well as check for beneficial bacteria.

In some rare cases, anxiety may originate in the stomach rather than the brain. Candidiasis, a gastrointestinal yeast infection, affects anxiety in about 5 percent of my patients. A simple stool sample identifies the type of yeast present (they are not all the same), as well as the antimicrobial that will eliminate it. This type of infection seems to make the infected person more susceptible to foods and chemicals, so it is helpful to eradicate it.

A number of scientists have suggested that up to 80 percent of the human immune system resides in the gastrointestinal tract—and immune strength has an impact on emotional stability. Almost everyone knows that beneficial bacteria (acidophilus, for example) defend the gut against foreign bacteria. Therefore, we can learn something about the immune system by a laboratory analysis of the gastrointestinal tract. Another benefit of this test is its ability to assess the gut's digestion and absorption capabilities. Treatments are oral, for the most part, so these two functions influence treatment.

Antioxidant Status

Antioxidant vitamins, including E, C, and beta-carotene, have potential health-promoting properties. A laboratory test for antioxidant status (specifically the antioxidant glutathione) may tell your doctor that you need a specific nutrient.

When glutathione supplies are decreased in the gut, you are susceptible to food and chemical sensitivities, as well as to stress. Glutathione ingestion will reduce some of the symptoms of anxiety and panic such as rapid heartbeat and shortness of breath. While I don't believe this is a complete treatment for anxiety, it does have validity in certain people. Sometimes I simply instruct the patient to do a home clinical trial and take half a teaspoonful of glutathione powder (see page 143) during any stressful event that would precipitate anxiety. If taking the glutathione powder prevents or reverses the anxiety, then this clinical trial would have positive results.

Fatty Acid Analysis (Blood Biopsy)

In the early 1990s researchers at the Harvard Medical School research facility began the development of a test to determine fatty acid levels in human cell membranes. Initially, the test was used for congenitally compromised children with severe metabolic abnormalities. Nevertheless, this test was so helpful that it seemed useful to many other health conditions, including mental disorders.

Around the mid-1990s, Dr. Patricia Kane, a California Ph.D./nutritionist, advocated converting the test from a research tool to a clinical aid for practitioners. The idea was to treat adults based on the test results as well as children. I was one of the first doctors to work with her and probably the first to use this tool for anxiety patients.

The test has spurred new applications and now is a common clinical test (as opposed to a research tool). The test is still used primarily by alternative care physicians and provides extensive insight into the body's nutrition status, fatty acid balance, mitochondrial energy efficiency, peroxisomal efficiency (detoxification), internal respiration, and more. In a sense, the test represents a chemical CAT scan of our metabolism. Although imperfect, it is still a big step in analyzing for chemical imbalances primarily related to nutritional factors that have to do with cell health. Results of the test give a more exact list of deficiencies and excesses. The prescribing physician can determine necessary dietary supplements and a practical daily meal plan. Here, foods and natural dietary supplements combine in a well-organized program to correct imbalances. This test is not specific to any health disorder but it can be helpful to anxiety patients. (I've given references to this test in the Resources at the back of the book.)

SPECT Image Graphics

Another diagnostic test, SPECT (single photon emission computed tomography), falls into the field of nuclear medicine. With SPECT, small doses of special radioisotopes are used to study cerebral perfusion and activity of the brain. The word "perfusion" refers to the level of circulation that nourishes an area of the brain. The word "activity" in this context means the level of conversion of sugar to energy and that in return is referred to as the level of metabolism.

With SPECT, you lie on your back on a mobile table that has a special 3-D camera over it. A physician injects the radioactive isotope intravenously before the test. This isotope, called a radiotracer and which gives only a minute amount of radiation, then passes through the blood to the brain, where it is taken up by certain receptor sites in the nerves. As you lie on the table, a camera uses special crystals that detect where the radioisotope has gone. The camera moves around the head, acting as a tracking device that tells where the blood flowed and where the most active cells are. The camera also detects where the least blood flowed and where the least active cells were at the time of the injection. A computer takes snapshots and reconstructs 3-D images of the whole brain, including exquisitely fine details of every area in the brain. This tells us if everything is all right, or if there is a problem and where it is located.

Both CAT scans and MRIs are superior to SPECT in regard to clarity of static anatomy. These two scans are better than SPECT when it comes to tumors, cysts, and blood clots. Yet they fall short of SPECT when it comes to imaging the real-time activity inside a working brain. While neurologists find great use in the CAT, MRI, and EEG studies, psychiatrists find that making a diagnosis is greatly improved with the SPECT scan.

With SPECT technology, we can make full-color images of the brain in action. We can see the parts of the brain that are working, the parts that are not working, and the areas that are overworking. We know what a normal brain should look like and we can measure how far away from normal the imaged brain might be. Then, we can see in a follow-up study the level of improvement following a regimen of proper nutrients or medications. We can view an unbalanced brain rebalancing itself during treatment. We now have tangible proof that something was wrong and then tangible proof that we have added agents (nutritional or medications) that brought it back toward a more normal appearance. This technology has been of great help to thousands of people with severe anxiety and no resolution to their problem.

Physicians who do SPECT scans have an entire formulary of natural dietary supplements they can apply to any involved area of the brain instead of drugs. Examples of the types of nutrients used include St. John's wort, 5-HTP, tryptophan, vitamin E, pine bark extract, amino acids, gingko biloba, gotu kola, omega-3 and omega-6 fatty acids, inositol, choline, and melatonin, among others.

The SPECT scan approach is on the cutting edge of medicine and in the early stages of maturation. For this reason, there are plenty of voices raised in criticism of the incomplete lack of science behind the technology. As always, leaders in the field will have to persevere against the opposition until the science catches up.

Who Benefits from SPECT?

- Anyone with stress, tension, or anxiety that has eluded satisfactory therapy after a reasonable number of attempts.
- Anxious students or workers who have difficulty learning—learning disabilities might be treatable once uncovered by SPECT.
- Those who are anxious and frustrated because they know they are performing below their potential.

- People with one of the difficult-to-diagnose forms of attention deficit disorder (ADD).
- Those with a nervous feeling following any type of head trauma.
- Older adults who are becoming more impatient or easily set off.
- Older adults who are becoming more frightened.

TESTING IS THE FIRST STEP TO LIVING ANXIETY-FREE

The outlook for people with anxiety disorders is remarkably better than ever before. Ongoing research and clinical trials are providing new information on the illness and how to treat successfully the variations in symptoms. However, before you can treat the symptoms, you must understand all you can about your illness. That's why a close-knit relationship with your doctor is vital in finding a treatment that really works.

This chapter discussed the basic laboratory tests and imaging scans both conventional and alternative medicine doctors use to diagnose anxiety disorders. While there are far too many variances of these tests to discuss all of them in this book, talk openly with your doctor to gain a full understanding before you agree to any test. Ask questions about what to expect during the test and if there are any precautions you should take. Also, seek a second opinion if you feel uncomfortable with the diagnosis or suggestions made by your doctor.

No matter what type of anxiety you have, aggressively work with your doctor to discover treatment modalities that resolve it so you can feel anxiety-free and regain your productive life.

‿‿

Chapter 6

Step 2: Start with Natural Therapies

"I will do anything to get well, but I don't want to take another medication." Lauren, a thirty-two-year-old magazine editor, was determined to avoid medications to help ease her panic attacks. "When I take drugs, my anxiety does ease some. But medications leave me feeling so numb and fatigued that I cannot function. So, what's the point?"

Hank, a forty-three-year-old CPA, knows all about anxiety disorders and the side effects of harsh medications. While anti-anxiety medications such as Xanax helped to calm his racing mind and stay asleep at night, they also made him drowsy and upset his gastrointestinal system, causing constipation and increased appetite.

Then Hank started taking the natural dietary supplement SAM-e, which is thought to raise levels of the neurotransmitter dopamine—vital for mood regulation. He continued the recommended program of vitamins and minerals to fortify his body and took a 3 mg capsule of melatonin before bedtime to aid in sleep. After seven days of taking SAM-e, Hank reported a dramatic improvement in his ability to think clearly along with reduced anxiety.

I cannot promise that every patient who takes SAM-e or other dietary supplements will have dramatic results like Hank. However, I do know that many nutrients can safely support a weakened immune system. We doctors know that when the immune system functions optimally, hormones are balanced and healing sleep is increased; as a result, overall anxiety is reduced sufficiently.

NATURAL THERAPIES FOR ANXIETY

While conventional medical doctors focus on defining disease based on symptoms and then eliminating those signs, alternative medical doctors strive to treat the whole person—body, mind, and spirit—with the focus on staying balanced and well. Most alternative modalities, which range from natural dietary supplements to lifestyle changes to mind-body exercises, are safe, effective, relatively affordable, and may allow you to participate actively in key decisions about your health.

By now, you know that I am a firm believer in strengthening the body naturally as the best way to reduce mild anxiety. In more severe anxiety cases, nutrients and lifestyle changes are not enough to give relief. That's why it is important to talk with your doctor and get an accurate medical diagnosis of your anxiety disorder before taking any new medication or alternative therapies. Although the natural dietary supplements described in this step may not be appropriate for your specific anxiety disorder, they have allowed thousands of my patients to regain control of their anxiety—and their lives.

Today in the United States, natural dietary supplements include a wide assortment of products, including multivitamins, minerals, amino acids, herbs, as well as ingredients derived from plant and animal sources. These are available in an assortment of forms from capsules, pills, and gel tabs, to liquids, tinctures, extracts, and powders.

Each month there are hundreds of new scientific papers related to natural dietary supplements. And those of us in the alternative medicine field thrive on these publications. Ironically, however, when a positive nutritional effect is discovered and published in a prestigious journal, the author suggests that a drug be developed mimicking this nutrient's effect. The value of the nutrient itself is ignored, while the value of its effect becomes the objective of a new drug, reflecting the values of the scientific research community, which relies heavily on funding from big drug companies. Nevertheless, like other alternative care providers, I pore over these same medical studies and use the very science to create natural therapies that drug companies use to create new pharmaceuticals.

Be Selective

When used properly, natural dietary supplements can safely, naturally, and effectively strengthen the body, and thus provide powerful relief from many types of mild anxiety. Still, it's important to educate yourself on how to choose the best brands.

Brand-name companies (this usually means they have been around for a long time and you recognize them) are almost always dependable because they are under more scrutiny by regulators. There is nothing wrong, however, with using products from smaller companies who often have the more unique formulas.

Natural dietary supplements vary in price depending on where they are purchased, how they are processed, and the strength of the ingredients. Some of your more expensive brands standardize their ingredients and use only organic products. If the ingredients are not standardized, the supplement may provide too little—or even too much—of the active ingredient.

Products keep coming at you from all directions and it would be hard for anyone to know who to trust and what to believe. If you are already acquainted with the nutritional field then you probably don't need much advice, but if you are new then do this: Use this book as a starting point to understand products and ideas and then gradually expand. Along the way you will develop a loyalty to a person or a group that will become your mentor. One of the websites where I write the newsletter on anxiety and depression is www.anxietyanddepressionrelief.com. There will be links from there to other nutritionally related sites.

In addition, read the supplement label carefully and notice the expiration date. Like any food product, supplements lose potency over time. If a supplement does not have an expiration date, be wary and do not buy it. And remember, virtually all nutritional products are required to have seals on the outside over the cap and on the inside after the cap has been removed. If you do not find these, then return the item.

Questions to Consider Before Taking a Natural Dietary Supplement

No matter what the supplement label claims about safety, the ingredients have not been tested nor does the FDA regulate them. That's why I encourage you to *talk with your doctor* before taking any supplement. Even natural supplements can cause serious, life-threatening symptoms or dangerous interactions with other supplements or medications. Herbal therapies are not recommended for pregnant women, children, the elderly, or those with compromised immune systems.

Consider the following questions before you take any unregulated product:

- Are there potential side effects?
- Can it interact with any foods?
- Can it interact with other medications or supplements?
- Is there sufficient scientific evidence that it is safe?
- Is this a reputable brand?

Alternative Therapies Take Time

While popular supplements such as valerian or SAM-e might work in just days, it often takes up to three months before some nutrients deliver the full effect; for that reason I often prescribe a pharmaceutical in the beginning of a patient's treatment. However, most of my patients report some benefit during the first week or so on the natural formulas.

Trial and Error

"But how will I know for sure if natural therapies work for me? I'd hate to be a long-term guinea pig when taking unknown therapies." Forty-one-year-old Macy approached natural therapies with some apprehension.

The way you will know which natural therapy works best for you is simple—by trial and error. In my practice, I ask patients to be part of a clinical trial to nail down the best nutrient. Clinical trial in this case means taking the nutrient home and trying it on for fit. A partial fit is good; but a perfect fit is terrific!

DR. HUNT'S HOLISTIC RX

In the upcoming pages, I will outline a nutrient supplement program for the common anxiety disorders discussed in Chapters 2 and 3 (see list below). These nutrients, given in the chart that follows, are based on the typical protocols I recommend to my patients. Let me remind you that the information in Step 2 is to be considered part of an overall lifestyle approach to ending anxiety. In no way is it a substitute for a good therapist or other health care professional. Rather, it may provide you with some insight and useful ideas to consider as you seek to strengthen the body. It is imperative that you talk to your doctor first to make sure these therapies will work for your situation.

Common Anxiety Disorders

Generalized anxiety disorder (GAD)—constant or exaggerated worries about everyday life events, lasting at least six months.

Simple phobia—overwhelming and unreasonable fears of a place or thing.

Social phobia—unreasonable and disabling fear of scrutiny or embarrassment in public situations.

Panic disorder—repeated episodes of intense fear that strike often and without warning.

Agoraphobia—fear of being in places or situations that are potentially embarrassing.

Obsessive-compulsive disorder (OCD)—unwanted thoughts or compulsive behaviors that seem impossible to stop or control.

Acute stress reaction—symptoms that appear within minutes of a traumatic event and disappear within days (even hours).

Adjustment disorder—emotional or behavioral symptoms that occur because of a series of stresses.

Post-traumatic stress disorder (PTSD)—persistent symptoms that occur after experiencing or witnessing a traumatic event.

The following chart (pages 132–135) can help you to individualize your formula. You will see the nutrients related to the various forms of anxiety. Do not take an action until you read the text pages following the chart to see if a nutrient in a specific category applies to you. If you implusively use the entire formula you will be taking extra nutrients you may not need.

For example, the recommendation that vitamin C be taken by those with GAD applies *only* to individuals with environmental sensitivities. If you do not react to your environment, then skip the C. Read on and find the individual nutrients that apply only to you.

Essential Nutrients for Easing Anxiety

	Vitamins and Minerals	Antioxidants	B Vitamins	Bioflavonoids	Botanicals	Amino Acids	Other Natural Therapies
Generalized anxiety disorder (GAD)	50 mg zinc 1x daily 300 mg calcium 3x daily 300 mg magnesium 3x daily	400 mg glutathione 3x daily ¼ tsp liquid selenium before bedtime 2,000 mg vitamin C 2x daily	100 mg thiamine 3x daily 100 mg pyridoxine 1x daily 1,000 mg pantothenic acid 3x daily 2 mg folic acid 1x daily	1,000 mg quercetin 2x daily 200 mg bromelain 3x daily	4–6 sprays peppermint as needed 100 mg capsule valerian at bedtime or 100 mg passionflower once or twice in evening hours	500 mg L-tyrosine 3x daily (for depression) 100 mg L-theanine 2x daily for relaxation	50 mg 5-HTP 3x daily 400 mg SAM-e 4x daily (for depression) 3 mg melatonin 1 hour before bedtime
Simple phobia	300 mg calcium 3x daily 300 mg magnesium 3x daily	N/A	100 mg thiamine 3x daily 1,000 mg pantothenic acid 3x daily		4–6 sprays peppermint as needed	100 mg L-theanine 2x daily for relaxation	50 mg 5-HTP 3x daily 3 mg melatonin 1 hour before bedtime
Social phobia	300 mg calcium 3x daily 300 mg magnesium 3x daily	400 mg glutathione 3x daily 200 mcg selenium 2x daily	100 mg thiamine 3x daily 1,000 mg pantothenic acid 3x daily		4–6 sprays peppermint as needed	100 mg L-theanine 2x daily for relaxation	50 mg 5-HTP 3x daily 3 mg melatonin 1 hour before bedtime

Panic Disorder	300 mg magnesium 1x daily	400 mg glutathione 3x daily 200 mcg selenium 2x daily 2,000 mg vitamin C 2x daily	2 mg folic acid 1x daily 100 mg thiamine 3x daily 1,000 mg pantothenic acid 3x daily 1,000 mg inositol 3x daily		4–6 sprays peppermint as needed 100 mg capsule valerian at bedtime or 100 mg passionflower once or twice in evening hours	100 mg L-theanine 2x daily for relaxation	50 mg 5-HTP 3x daily 3 mg melatonin 1 hour before bedtime
Agoraphobia	300 mg calcium 3x daily 300 mg magnesium 3x daily	400 mg glutathione 3x daily 200 mcg selenium 2x daily 2,000 mg vitamin C 3x daily	100 mg thiamine 3x daily 1,000 mg pantothenic acid 3x daily 1 mg vitamin B$_{12}$ sublingually 1x daily 1,000 mg inositol 3x daily 2 mg folic acid 1x daily	1,000 mg quercetin 2x daily	4–6 sprays peppermint as needed 100 mg capsule valerian at bedtime or 100 mg passionflower once or twice in evening hours	100 mg L-theanine 2x daily for relaxation	50 mg 5-HTP 3x daily 3 mg melatonin 1 hour before bedtime

(continued)

Essential Nutrients for Easing Anxiety (*continued*)

	Vitamins and Minerals	Antioxidants	B Vitamins	Bioflavonoids	Botanicals	Amino Acids	Other Natural Therapies
Obsessive-compulsive disorder (OCD)		400 mg glutathione 3x daily	1,000 mg inositol 3x daily		4–6 sprays peppermint as needed	100 mg L-theanine 2x daily for relaxation	50 mg 5-HTP 3x daily 3 mg melatonin 1 hour before bedtime
Acute stress reaction					4–6 sprays peppermint as needed 100 mg capsule valerian at bedtime or 100 mg passionflower once or twice in evening hours	100 mg L-theanine 2x daily for relaxation	3 mg melatonin 1 hour before bedtime
Adjustment disorder		10,000 IU vitamin A 1x daily 200 mcg selenium 2x daily			4–6 sprays peppermint as needed	100 mg L-theanine 2x daily for relaxation	3 mg melatonin 1 hour before bedtime

Post-traumatic stress disorder (PTSD)		1 scoop glutathione in 1 cup water 200 mcg selenium 2x daily 400 mg vitamin E 2x daily	100 mg thiamine 3x daily 1 mg vitamin B_{12} sublingually 1x daily		4–6 sprays peppermint as needed 100 mg capsule valerian at bedtime or 100 mg passionflower once or twice in evening hours	100 mg L-theanine 2x daily for relaxation	50 mg 5-HTP 3x daily 3 mg melatonin 1 hour before bedtime
	400 mg vitamin E 2x daily						

VITAMINS AND MINERALS

Vitamins are key for normal metabolism, growth, mental alertness, and chronic disease prevention. These chemically unrelated families of organic substances are divided into two categories:

1. Water-soluble, which dissolve in water and are not absorbed by the body in large amounts. Excess water-soluble vitamins are excreted in urine.
2. Fat-soluble, which are absorbed in body fat and the liver. Excess fat-soluble vitamins can accumulate and be toxic.

Minerals act as building blocks for cells and enzymes and are the main components in teeth and bones. Serving as the regulators of the fluid balance in the body, minerals help deliver oxygen to cells and carry away carbon dioxide. They also control the movement of nerve impulses.

While a nutrient-dense diet rich in vitamins and minerals plays a key role in strengthening the body and preventing disease, researchers have targeted specific vitamins and minerals that might influence anxiety disorders. There are no guarantees that these will work for everyone, but I do know that these nutrients help most of my patients increase their get-up-and-go and boost immune function. And, as I've said before, when you experience optimal health, you sleep better, feel alert and energetic, and handle life's stressors more effectively.

Calcium

Calcium is a wonder mineral, as it influences many of the body's functions. Study after study confirms that a diet high in calcium helps to ward off osteoporosis or brittle bones. Evidence also suggests that calcium plays a key role in your emotional health, specifically for the speed and efficiency of neurotransmitter transmission. In a sense, calcium acts like a gatekeeper in that many neurotransmitter impulses must pass through a calcium channel located in a nerve cell wall.

Some research indicates that dietary calcium may help lower blood pressure, which can be raised during times of anxiety. This key mineral is important for muscle contraction and communication between nerve cells—all vital in supporting the body during anxiety and panic.

I recommend taking 300 mg of calcium three times a day for generalized anxiety disorder, social phobia, and agoraphobia. Calcium supplementation works best when combined with magnesium (see below). Body Relief, a blend of calcium, magnesium, and vitamin B_1 in capsule form, is available at www.anxietyanddepressionrelief.com. Many of my patients who take Body Relief appreciate the convenience of this product.

To get ample calcium in the diet, eat plenty of broccoli, bok choy, salmon, sardines with bones, kale, beans (dried), dairy products, soy products, and calcium-fortified foods.

Magnesium

Magnesium is a power mineral that has many beneficial effects on anxiety. Not only is magnesium a muscle relaxer, it is a natural remedy to calm the sympathetic nervous system (SNS), which mediates the body's fight-or-flight response to stressful situations. Magnesium is also involved in essential fatty acid metabolism, dopamine production, and insulin secretion.

Some interesting research reported in the *Journal of the American College of Nutrition* found that low blood and tissue levels of magnesium during times of emotional or other stress could produce extreme levels of anxiety and depression. Low levels of magnesium increase the release of catecholamines. Catecholamines are hormones, including epinephrine and norepinephrine, that influence blood sugar levels, which, in turn, lower heart magnesium levels. This physiologic state results in excess release or formation of vascular factors that are vasoconstrictive (narrowing of the opening of a blood vessel) and clot-forming (platelet aggregating). Dietary imbalances caused by high fat or calcium intake can be harmful because they intensify a preexisting magnesium deficiency.

When blood magnesium levels drop, your body's adrenaline levels soar, resulting in a nervous system on high alert. The rush of adrenaline is poison to an already anxious person. Low magnesium levels, in addition, allow the body's insulin levels to climb high enough to create fatigue and hypoglycemia or low blood sugar, physical states unhelpful to the anxious person.

I recommend taking 300 mg of magnesium three times a day for generalized anxiety disorder, simple phobia, social phobia, panic disorder, agoraphobia, or any other form of anxiety in which the physical symptoms are more than mild. The product Body Relief contains the mineral magnesium, properly balanced with calcium, and is available at www.anxietyanddepression.com. To get plenty of magnesium in your diet, eat cereal, nuts, sunflower seeds, tofu, dairy products, bananas, pineapple, plantains, raisins, artichokes, avocados, lima beans, spinach, okra, beet greens, hummus, oysters, halibut, mackerel, grouper, cod, and sole.

Zinc

Zinc is an essential mineral for good health, keeping your immune system actively fighting viruses and bacteria and helping to support healthy growth and development. Remember, a healthy body functions optimally and helps you cope with daily stressors.

I recommend taking 50 mg of zinc once a day for generalized anxiety disorder, especially for those who have a tendency toward frequent respiratory infections. To get plenty of zinc in the diet, eat meat, pork, poultry, seafood, wheat products, nuts, seeds, dairy products, and zinc-fortified products.

ANTIOXIDANTS

Some nutrients, called antioxidants, are cleansing agents intimately involved in the prevention of cellular damage—the common pathway for cancer, aging, and a variety of diseases. These nutrients build immunity and are cofactors in the creation of most neurotransmitters, key brain chemicals. Cofactors are the additional secondary nutrients that are essential for a biochemical enzymatic reaction to occur. No nutrient functions alone; they must have collaborating nutrients for the enzymes to work. Enzymes that expedite chemical changes require a minimum of at least one vitamin and one mineral before they can activate. When you are stressed to the point that you become relatively deficient in nutrients, then your neurotransmitter supplies will be deficient as well.

In addition, human cell membranes (including nerve cells), which are mostly composed of essential fats (and thus vulnerable to rancidity), are severely threatened when there is an increase in free radicals, emanating from a stressful experience. Free radicals are highly charged particles that reverberate wildly and damage cell structures making them vulnerable to decay and pathogens. Cell walls will begin to lose their permeability and become rigid and nonfunctional when bombarded by these destructive particles.

If not removed, the free radicals or metabolic wastes become toxic to our normal biochemistry and even our tissues. High levels of free radicals produce harmful short- and long-term symptoms as well as organic damage. Emotional symptoms of free radical damage include hyperactivity, nervous tension, anxiety, and restlessness. Physical damage caused by free radicals is thought to be the basic mechanism behind aging, atherosclerosis, cancer, rheumatic diseases, allergies, inflammation, and a host of other problems.

Because antioxidants are known to neutralize free radicals, the obvious solution would be an antioxidant to help protect and even heal the body. Along with vitamins A, C, and E, and selenium, clinical experience indicates that one of the best antioxidants for a mental problem is glutathione or GSH, a multitasking antioxidant of monumental proportions.

In findings published in the January 2003 issue of the *Journal of Biology and Chemistry,* researchers concluded that glutathione is necessary to activate production of the brain chemical dopamine under conditions of oxidative stress and/or drug-induced toxicity. In other findings published in 2002 in the journal of *Neuropsychobiology,* researchers found that free radicals were associated with some symptoms of obsessive-compulsive disorder as well as other types of anxiety. This same team of researchers undertook a similar experiment the year before and linked panic disorder with free radical damage.

When we entertain the subject of free radicals, we have automatically entered the arena of mitochondria, tiny little energy packs (dots) that inhabit every cell in our body. Mito-chondria make the energy that runs your body and plays a key role in mental health. There are approximately 300 mito-chondria in an average cell, but there are 10,000 to every heart muscle cell.

Mitochondria are the main source of free radicals in the body. The reactive molecules (free radicals) may damage any cellular part, especially DNA, membranes, and proteins, in-cluding components in the mitochondria itself. Damaged mitochondria will accumulate and get in the way of other mi-tochondria. This is considered a cause of tissue aging by inter-fering with the optimal energy machinery.

When GSH is missing or greatly decreased, there is often severe damage to the mitochondrial system within cells. If the mitochondrial health fails over time, the free radicals increase exponentially. Conversely, when the mitochondria improve, free radicals decline, along with subsequent damage to the mind and body.

Damaged mitochondria decrease cellular bioenergetic ca-pacity. This increases the generation of reactive oxygen species (free radicals), resulting in oxidative damage and programmed cell death. This dangerous cycle never ends. Our cellular mi-tochondrial efficiency directly affects the level of energy we feel. It is obvious then that inefficient, dysfunctional, or dam-aged mitochondria result in fatigue, and, again, fatigue is an instigator of anxiety.

Inefficient mitochondria produce many symptoms when there are significant numbers of them in trouble. These in-clude arrhythmias, sudden rapid heartbeats, periods of breath-lessness, and abrupt rushes of fear with and without a full panic attack.

The bottom line is that mitochondrial efficiency prevents

fatigue—and that should be your goal when adding antioxidants to your daily nutrients.

Mitochondria are absolutely necessary for energy, stamina, physical strength, and even life itself. It takes only a slight drop in the mitochondrial energy output to result in bodily weakness and emotional and physical fatigue. Aging as well as stress compromises mitochondrial efficiency.

Virtually every common nutrient will strengthen the mitochondria, but some are more helpful than others. Surprisingly, the B vitamins are some of the best supporters, followed by the amino acid carnitine and coenzyme Q10.

Vitamin A. Vitamin A, a fat-soluble vitamin that is stored in the body, is a super-antioxidant that is important for immune function, building strong bones, cell division, and more.

I recommend taking 10,000 international units (IU) of vitamin A daily for adjustment disorders and any stress related to the environment. Liver and eggs contain retinal, a usable form of vitamin A, and colorful fruits and vegetables contain carotenoids that the liver converts to retinal. Beta-carotene is the molecule that gives carrots and sweet potatoes their bright orange color.

Vitamin C. Vitamin C (otherwise known as ascorbic acid), is the most abundant water-soluble antioxidant in the body. Vitamin C must be replenished to keep your immune system functioning normally.

Vitamin C also helps to boost levels of the energizing brain chemical norepinephrine, which produces a feeling of alertness and increases concentration. This is especially important for those with anxiety who experience periods of inattentiveness.

I recommend taking 2,000 mg of vitamin C twice daily for generalized anxiety disorder, panic disorder, agoraphobia, or any other form of anxiety that is triggered or worsened by an allergy or sensitivity to environmental chemicals, pollens, foods, molds, or pet dander. You can get plenty of vitamin C by eating broccoli, cauliflower, peppers, kale, Brussels sprouts, cabbage, citrus fruit, melons, asparagus, avocados, kohlrabi, mustard greens, tomatoes, and watercress.

Vitamin E. Vitamin E is the most abundant fat-soluble antioxidant in the body and is crucial for the maintenance of cell membranes. Vitamin E may slow age-related changes in the body.

I recommend taking 400 mg of vitamin E twice daily for adjustment disorder and post-traumatic stress disorder. Eat plenty of cold-pressed seeds and oils, wheat germ, nuts, mango, pumpkin, and green leafy vegetables like broccoli, chard, kohlrabi, spinach, and greens of dandelion, mustard, and turnip. You can find vitamin E in meat, fish, poultry, clams, mackerel, lobster, salmon, and shrimp.

Glutathione. As mentioned, this antioxidant performs a wide variety of physiological and metabolic tasks, not least of which is its ability to preserve tissue integrity.

I recommend taking 400 mg of glutathione powder three times a day for social phobia, panic disorder, agoraphobia, obsessive-compulsive disorder, and post-traumatic stress disorder. It may also benefit anyone with generalized anxiety disorder, especially if there is a great deal of stress. Eat foods rich in glutathione such as broccoli, asparagus, cabbage, cauliflower, potatoes, and tomatoes. Fruits with glutathione include avocados, grapefruit, oranges, peaches, and watermelon.

Selenium. Selenium is an important trace mineral that may hold the key to staying disease-free, as it helps to keep the immune system working optimally and is important for a healthy thyroid gland. Selenium functions as an antioxidant, as it helps to fight free radicals that cause damage to healthy tissue. Selenium demonstrates antiviral activity by increasing T-lymphocytes and enhancing the activity of natural killer cells—all important for optimal immune function and disease prevention.

I recommend taking 200 micrograms of selenium twice daily for panic disorder, agoraphobia, adjustment disorder, post-traumatic stress disorder, or any form of anxiety in which there is sensitivity to chemicals, severe current stress, or clear elevation of excitement. The preferred form of selenium is liquid sodium selenite. Eat plenty of Brazil nuts, beef, tuna, turkey, chicken, walnuts, cheese, eggs, cottage cheese, and grain products.

Alice's Feeling of Impending Doom

When I first met Alice, age forty-one, she said she felt anxious and apathetic, even when she was with friends or family. This bright, attractive woman said there was a feeling of impending doom all the time, even when she had no real problems to consider. Alice went on to tell about finishing her MBA, some upcoming interviews with corporate powerhouses, and how her son was voted president of his senior class. While she had so much to be excited about, she said she didn't have that optimistic feeling inside like she used to have.

I suggested that Alice start taking SAM-e, along with glutathione and folic acid. Within one week, her mood changed from cynical and negative to upbeat and enthusiastic again. Alice said she slept better than she had in years and started looking forward to all the upcoming events in her life.

B VITAMINS

We doctors know that during stress there is a significant loss of B vitamins through the urinary system. The urinary loss of water-soluble B vitamins is because of the elevation of gluco-corticoids released by the adrenal gland, which is attempting to adapt to the stress.

Bs Boost the Body

I use B vitamins along with the antioxidants to boost the body during stressful times. For example, the B vitamin thiamine (B_1) is a valuable nutrient for anyone who harbors the physical form of anxiety. Because thiamine is not stored in the body, it must be supplied in the daily diet. If you eat adequate amounts of unprocessed whole grains, there is no problem. However, the consumption of high-calorie, low-nutrient junk foods can cause a depletion of vitamins, especially the water-soluble Bs such as thiamine and vitamin B_6. Table sugar, sweets, nicotine, caffeine, and alcohol are also destructive to this nutrient.

Balancing the Hypothalamus

The hypothalamus, the area of the brain that controls neuro-logical stability, has the power to switch our feelings on and off. It is just as vulnerable to malnutrition, including marginal malnutrition, as any other part of the brain. If thiamine is de-pleted in the sympathetic part of the hypothalamus, there will be increased activity in the sympathetic nervous system, pro-ducing excitement and nervousness. When thiamine is in-gested, the sympathetic nervous system quiets down again and the person becomes calm, relaxed, and free of tension.

If thiamine (vitamin B$_1$) is over-utilized by the hypothalamus during stressful times, a deficiency of this vitamin can occur. During the initial thiamine-deficiency stage, it is not uncommon to have symptoms of anxiety, irritability, fatigue, depression, and personality changes. Before the physical symptoms develop, such emotional changes are often dismissed as purely psychological in origin. Thiamine deficiency also decreases cell energy and that adds to the symptom mix.

The Thiamine-Anxiety Connection

Some patients with clinical thiamine deficiencies have symptoms similar to panic attacks, including sleep disturbances, nausea, tendency to sweat, chronic depression, dizziness, and recurring infections. One of the first signs of a thiamine deficiency is an unstable autonomic nervous system, the system that modulates blood pressure. Many of these patients exhibit unstable blood pressure, ticlike movements, neurological reflex disturbances, and abdominal and chest pains.

The hypothalamus can become overloaded by any excessive stress such as chronic mononucleosis, extended grief, or an overdose of an anesthetic. The hypothalamus will make a valiant attempt to maintain control, of course, but if the assault is excessive, the organ can fail. Since thiamine is important to the hypothalamus, even the slightest deficit will affect its efficiency. Thiamine metabolism in the hypothalamus may never really catch up to its needs if the deficiency is too great. This is also true if the unlucky individual has inherited a genetic flaw that causes improper reactions to stress. A person weakened by a genetic mistake will be overwhelmed and may not bounce back.

With thiamine, reinstating a normal balance may take months, even years. It's easy to see why susceptible people seem to take forever to recover. Stress-vulnerable people require high levels of nutrition both during and after stress; otherwise, they will continue to have borderline health.

B₁ (Thiamine). Thiamine is an important enzyme in the body, as it metabolizes sugar and supports the nervous system. This nutrient also is connected to muscular strength, involved in constructing neurotransmitters, important to immune strength, and is a critical agent in energy generation. One of the first symptoms of a thiamine deficiency is anxiety.

I recommend 100 mg of thiamine three times a day for generalized anxiety disorder, phobias, panic disorder, agoraphobia, obsessive-compulsive disorder, and post-traumatic stress disorder. Please note that the amount of thiamine present in most multivitamins that contain B vitamins is insufficient and should be supplemented. You can get plenty of thiamine by eating wheat germ, peanuts, peas, liver, legumes, and cereal grains.

Vitamin B₅ (Pantothenic Acid). Vitamin B₅ or pantothenic acid is a main ingredient in brewer's yeast, a popular supplement taken to boost energy. This important vitamin is a key nutrient for neuroprotection.

I recommend taking 1,000 mg of pantothenic acid (B₅) three times a day for generalized anxiety disorder, all types of phobias, panic disorder, agoraphobia, and any form of anxiety that worsens with an immune weakness such as excessive allergies. Eat plenty of brewer's or nutritional yeast, whole grain breads and cereals, dried beans, avocados, fish, chicken, liver, nuts (pecans, hazelnuts), peanuts, cauliflower, mushrooms, potatoes, oranges, bananas, milk and cheese, and eggs.

Vitamin B₆ (Pyridoxine). Pyridoxine, a water-soluble B vitamin, works as a cofactor in more than 100 enzyme reactions, particularly those related to the metabolism of amino acids and other proteins. Pyridoxine affects the synthesis of serotonin and dopamine, neurotransmitters necessary for healthy nerve cell communication (pages 86–90). Symptoms of deficiency may include depression, irritability, and premenstrual syndrome (PMS).

I recommend taking 100 mg of pyridoxine (B_6) once a day for generalized anxiety disorder because of its benefits to the neurotransmitters. You can get B_6 by eating chicken, fish, liver, kidney, pork, bananas, spinach, sweet potatoes, white potatoes, garbanzo beans, walnuts, brown rice, soybeans, sunflower seeds, avocados, oats, peanuts, lima beans, peanut butter, prunes, and whole wheat products.

Vitamin B_{12} (Cobalamin). If you are a meat eater, then getting enough vitamin B_{12} is probably not a problem. This important vitamin—tagged the "energy vitamin"—is found in meat, fish, eggs, and dairy products. Vegetarians are at high risk for B_{12} deficiency, which can be measured by a blood test.

I recommend taking 1 mg of vitamin B_{12} once a day for agoraphobia, post-traumatic stress disorder, or any other form of anxiety where lack of energy or depression is making the anxiety worse. I suggest using a sublingual (under the tongue) form of vitamin B_{12} such as a liquid or a lozenge. To get adequate B_{12}, eat plenty of meat, fish, eggs, dairy products, and nutritional or brewer's yeast.

Folic acid. Folic acid and folate are forms of the water-soluble B vitamin. Folate occurs naturally in food. Folic acid is the synthetic form found in fortified foods and dietary supplements. Research shows there is a high incidence of folate deficiency in depression, and clinical studies indicate that some depressed patients who are folate-deficient respond to folate administration.

I recommend taking 2 mg of folic acid once a day for generalized anxiety disorder, social phobia, agoraphobia, and any other form of anxiety where there is a hormonal or mood relationship. To get folate naturally, eat fortified breakfast cereals, wheat germ, spinach, oranges, broccoli, asparagus, beets, spinach, turnip greens, cabbage, egg yolks, turkey, cowpeas, chick peas, lentils, black beans, kidney beans, and soybeans.

Inositol. Comprehensive studies have been done over the years on the link between inositol and anxiety. For example, in a study published in the July 1995 issue of *The American Journal of Psychiatry,* twenty-one patients suffering from panic disorder completed a four-week treatment trial using 12 grams of inositol daily. The frequency and severity of the panic attacks dropped significantly during this time. The authors concluded that since the side effects were minimal, the product was natural, and the response was good, this form of treatment should be considered as a potentially viable therapy.

The authors began another test in which thirteen patients diagnosed with obsessive-compulsive disorder were given 18 grams of inositol daily for six weeks. At the end, the Obsessive Compulsive Scale tests were clearly much lower than the starting scores taken six weeks before. The authors concluded that inositol should be considered an effective treatment for depression, panic, and OCD symptoms. These three problems represent a spectrum of disorders that are responsive to selective serotonin reuptake inhibitors or SSRIs.

Another group of scientists decided to compare inositol's benefits to those of fluvoxamine (Luvox), a prescription drug known to be effective for panic disorder. In the findings published in the June 2001 issue of *Journal of Clinical Psychopharmacology,* twenty patients were placed on 18 grams of inositol daily for four weeks, and then on fluvoxamine, 150 mg daily for a month. The number of panic attacks per week dropped by 4 during the inositol period and by 2.4 in the fluvoxamine period. The other difference noted was that the fluvoxamine treatment produced some degree of nausea and fatigue, but natural therapy with inositol did not. The authors urged scientists to try to reproduce these results so that the medical community might accept this therapy in mainstream practice. Unfortunately, that is not likely to happen because the outcome would not result in profits for the drug companies, but would further support alternative care proponents.

The average dose for inositol is 12 grams a day, but you have to work up to that dose gradually. The one side effect noticed is loose stools. If that occurs, drop the dose back slightly and keep it at that level.

I recommend a starting dose of 1,000 mg of inositol three times a day for panic disorder and obsessive-compulsive disorder. Gradually build up to 2 grams, three times a day, and slowly add until you reach 4 grams, three times a day (12 grams). Eat cereal, grains, legumes, and meat.

Eat to "B" Anxiety-Free

The following whole foods are the best way to ingest the B vitamins, along with other key nutrients:

Vitamin	Food Sources
B_1 (Thiamine)	Wheat germ, peanuts, peas
B_2 (Riboflavin)	Dairy products, broccoli, tuna, salmon

B_3 (Niacin)	Brewer's or nutritional yeast, poultry, eggs, peanuts
B_5 (Pantothenic acid)	Soybeans, liver, fish, bananas, oatmeal
B_6 (Pyridoxine)	Cheese, cauliflower, beans, sweet potatoes
B_{12} (Cobalamin)	Meat, fish, eggs, dairy, and brewer's or nutritional yeast (some brands)
Folic acid	Green leafy vegetables, beans, sweet potatoes, oranges

BIOFLAVONOIDS

Traditional practitioners typically ignore environmental triggers to anxiety. It's a mistake to do so because physical damage to the nervous system is taking place simultaneous to the nervous discomfort. In the case of chemicals, the most appropriate antioxidants are the bioflavonoids.

The plant-derived bioflavonoids, often found in combination with vitamin C, have strong antioxidant and anti-inflammatory properties and appear to modulate key enzyme reactions in the inflammatory cascade. Bioflavonoids are found in green tea, citrus fruit, berries, onions, and pitted fruits. Supplemental bioflavonoids are available, including rutin, quercetin, bromelain, hesperidin, and proanthocyanidins. All affect the structure of collagen, protecting it from free radical destruction and cross-linking directly with the collagen fibers.

Quercetin

Quercetin, or vitamin P, a water-soluble nutrient related to vitamin C, is a popular bioflavonoid. It is generally found in plants that contain vitamin C. Quercetin's most useful effect in anxiety is to reduce environmental allergy sensitivities that trigger anxiety. Long-term use of quercetin may serve to reduce the body's reactiveness to foods or pollens.

I recommend taking 1,000 mg of quercetin two times a day for generalized anxiety disorder, agoraphobia, and any form of anxiety that is triggered by food or pollen sensitivities. Food sources of quercetin include onions, apples, and buckwheat.

Bromelain

Bromelain is a natural protein-digesting enzyme found in pineapple that has an anti-inflammatory effect. It is commonly used as a digestive aid and is often found in products designed to alleviate gastrointestinal discomfort.

I recommend taking 200 mg of bromelain three times a day for generalized anxiety disorder, especially when gastrointestinal discomfort exacerbates the anxiety. Food sources of bromelain include pineapple.

BOTANICALS

Herbs or botanicals work by directly interacting with the body chemistry. Some herbs are ingested through the mouth and to the bloodstream via the digestive system. Others are rubbed onto the skin and then move into the bloodstream.

The whole herb consists of the entire plant processed into

liquid or capsule form. Some herbs are in capsules made from a whole herb or extract. These are easiest to store and are available at most grocery, drug, or natural food stores. Herbs also come in liquids, either a tincture (made from the whole herb) or an extract (made from one or more parts of the herb). Herbs that are in a liquid are usually more potent.

Essential Oils

Aromatherapists have long supported the idea that essential oils (EOs) have a major impact either as calming agents or mild stimulants. These various plant-derived oils have been used traditionally to treat mental disorders. One particularly useful EO is peppermint oil, which is believed to possess psychoactive actions, particularly in reversing mental fatigue. In findings published in the July/August 2001 issue of the journal *Pharmacology Biochemistry and Behavior*, researchers injected peppermint oil into mice and concluded that their ambulatory activity increased dramatically. The authors broke out the constituent chemicals in peppermint oil and tested them separately. Most of them were as active as the oil itself.

Powerful Peppermint

Peppermint or menthol comes from the mint family of plants, *Lamiaceae*. Typically, it can be purchased as a tea, an extract, or in oil-containing capsules. Peppermint is an extract of the leaves and flowering tops of the plant *Mentha piperita*. More than a hundred different chemical components are extracted from the plant, but the main one is menthol.

Peppermint is a powerful calcium channel blocker and so it can be utilized in that capacity. Calcium channel blockers

(CCBs) are a group of drugs that interfere with the actions of calcium. Blocking calcium channels in cell walls has been found to have many benefits, including diminishing anxiety.

Most of the scientific studies, and there are dozens, have involved the gastrointestinal tract. Peppermint has been found useful in alleviating irritable bowel syndrome, colitis, H pylori infections, ulcers, indigestion, and gas; as an anti-emetic and digestive aid; and even in the treatment of gastrointestinal cancer.

The effect of a locally applied peppermint oil preparation was tested on tension-type headaches. In a German study published in the August 1996 issue of the journal *Nervenarzt,* 10 percent peppermint oil in ethanol was applied across the forehead and temples of patients of both sexes, ages eighteen to sixty-five. A total of 164 headaches were studied. Comparisons were made to the effects of 1,000 mg of acetaminophen (Tylenol) as well as to a placebo. The authors found that peppermint oil was working in fifteen minutes, but so was the acetaminophen, so the effect was about equal. When the two analgesics were used together, the effect was stronger than either used alone, and as a bonus there were no reported side effects.

In another similar study published in the September 1997 issue of *Journal of Advanced Nursing,* a British researcher studied the effects of peppermint oil on post-operative nausea in a group of gynecological patients. The researcher found that peppermint oil relieved the nausea and stress of the condition and the cost of the nutritional treatment was a pittance compared to the traditional anti-nausea drugs.

I started prescribing peppermint for stress headaches because several studies had proven it to be effective. Then, a serendipitous event occurred. Patients who took the oil to avoid headaches began reporting that it also stopped their panic attacks and obsessive worrying. I was so encouraged that I began using it for other forms of fear, panic, and anxiety. In my practice, this treatment continues to work far beyond my early expectations.

The most common form of peppermint is in enteric-coated capsules, but peppermint oil is also available in teas, tinctures, and in one-ounce dropper bottles.

Peppermint oil will take care of almost any phobia that is below the extreme level. It works well for fears involving public speaking, travel, animals, dentists, doctors, and confrontations. Therefore, peppermint oil is effective for panic as well as all mild to moderate levels of phobias and even some severe cases.

I recommend 4 to 6 puffs of peppermint spray (listed in Resources as the product Body Control) as needed to terminate a panic attack or to resolve any type of anxiety. Substitutes might include 2 capsules of peppermint, a cup of peppermint tea, or 25 drops of tincture of peppermint dissolved in water.

Ginseng

Ginseng boosts the immune response by increasing the number of antibodies in the body. Ginseng stimulates memory, counteracts fatigue, and soothes damage caused by stress. It may also increase stamina and well-being. Unlike other natural stimulants, ginseng acts without negative side effects such as irritability, addiction, and anxiety.

I recommend taking 2 or 3 drops under the tongue of a Korean ginseng tincture (see Resources) as needed for calming daytime agitation or overcoming insomnia.

Valerian

The botanical valerian has a sedative effect and has been shown to help in relieving insomnia or disrupted sleep habits by calming nerves and easing nervous tension. Valerian is regarded as a mild tranquilizer and has been deemed safe by Commission E (Germany's equivalent of our FDA) for treating sleep disorders brought on by nervous conditions. Unlike prescription or over-the-counter sleep and anxiety medications, valerian is not habit-forming, nor does it produce a hangover-like side effect.

I recommend taking one 100 mg valerian capsule or 10 drops valerian tincture in water as needed for insomnia. Sometimes I have the patient take one valerian capsule, once or twice (several hours apart) before bedtime, to gradually reduce anxiety.

Passionflower

Passionflower has mild sedative properties and can help alleviate insomnia, stress, and anxiety. Findings reported in the July 2001 issue of the *Journal of Clinical Pharmacy and Therapeutics* concluded that passionflower might reduce muscle spasms— important for those who suffer with chronic muscle tension along with anxiety.

I use passionflower for insomnia the same way I use valerian. Sometimes I rotate the two botanicals so the nutrient does not result in a tolerance, which can happen with long-term or regular usage of any medication or alternative therapy. Tolerance means the body appears to benefit less and less from the therapeutic substance ingested. There are numerous causes for this phenomenon but there are some counter-therapies. One can take a vacation from the substance—a week, a month, or even longer—and then try it again. You can use the same substance but from a different manufacturer or find a substitute altogether. For example, cranberry juice has been useful for reducing bladder infections. If it begins to fail one can substitute blueberry juice because they are similar in chemistry but are different plants.

I recommend taking 100 mg of passionflower once or twice during the evening as needed for calming and to prepare for restful sleep.

AMINO ACIDS

Amino acids are supplied by protein and are the building blocks that build, repair, and maintain your body tissues. Nine of them are essential and come from our food supply because the body does not make them. Other amino acids are non-essential because the body makes them if you eat enough calories and amino acids each day. Besides building cells and repairing tissue, amino acids form antibodies to combat invading bacteria and viruses.

The word "essential" when used in medicine means the body is unable to create the essential substance within itself and must ingest it or a deficiency will develop. The word "nonessential" when related to a nutrient means the body can make it if it is not in the food eaten. Lately, a third term has appeared: "conditionally essential," meaning that from time to time, especially during stress, disease or during an extremely unbalanced diet a normally nonessential nutrient such as arginine becomes an essential nutrient because the body cannot keep up with the demand and so must now ingest arginine or develop deficiency symptoms. The line between an essential and nonessential nutrient is becoming more blurred.

During acute stress, glucocorticoids, such as the stress hormone cortisol, are produced and released by the adrenal gland cortex. These are used by the body to promote survival by mobilizing energy reserves and accentuating the adrenergic nervous system. While cortisol is essential for survival, it is only a good guy for a short time. After a few days or weeks, depending on the person, it may start to degrade many of the body's normal balances. At some point, an elevated cortisol level loses its beneficial effect and converts into a toxin. Cortisol has been implicated in depression. This very significant mood alteration confirms the damage to nerves inflicted by long-term exposure to excessive hormones.

L-tyrosine

Tyrosine is an important neurotransmitter precursor because it is transformed by the brain into the very important anti-anxiety neurotransmitter dopamine. Dopamine is quieting to the emotional system, and anxiety can occur when it's in short supply. SPECT scans (pages 121–124) suggest that dopamine may be associated with social phobia because social phobic people may have fewer brain dopamine receptors. Tyrosine is thought to ease depression caused by dopamine inefficiency.

I recommend taking 500 mg of the amino acid tyrosine three times a day to relieve any depression associated with generalized anxiety disorder.

L-theanine

L-theanine, a derivative of the amino acid L-glutamine, is a calming amino acid found in green tea that stimulates the near-sleep alpha waves in the brain. Dopamine, another brain chemical with mood-enhancing properties, is also increased by L-theanine. While L-theanine does not make you sleepy like some herbal calming ingredients, it does have mild sedating properties.

I recommend taking 100 mg of L-theanine twice a day for anxiety patients who seek relaxation. For those with post-traumatic stress disorder, I recommend taking 500 mg each of the amino acids L-lysine and L-arginine three times a day for one month to reduce anxiety.

Amino Acids

Essential Amino Acids	Function in the Body
L-leucine and Isoleucine	Keeps you alert, gives energy
L-lysine	Forms collagen, may be effective against herpes, aids in production of hormones
L-methionine	Prevents hair and skin problems, lowers cholesterol levels, protects kidneys
L-phenylalanine	Produces norepinephrine, keeps you alert, improves memory, reduces hunger
L-threonine	Aids digestive process, assists metabolism
L-tryptophan	Natural relaxant, alleviates insomnia. Helps in treatment of migraines
L-valine	Promotes mental alertness, calms emotions
Nonessential Amino Acids	**Function in the Body**
L-alanine	Energizes brain and central nervous system, strengthens immune function
L-arginine	Improves immune response, promotes wound healing, releases growth hormones
L-aspartate	Increases endurance, energizes
L-cystine	Antioxidant, slows aging process, stimulates wound healing
L-glutamine	Improves mental capabilities, controls cravings for sugar, energizes

Nonessential Amino Acids	Function in the Body (*continued*)
L-glycine	Boosts immune function
L-histidine	Helps heal allergic diseases, arthritis, ulcers, and anemia
L-proline	Maintains and strengthens heart muscles
L-serine	Strengthens immune system
L-taurine	Reduces changes of aging, clears free radical wastes
L-tyrosine	Overcomes depression, increases alertness, promotes healthy thyroid function

OTHER NATURAL THERAPIES

The following nutrients can be employed when they seem applicable. For example, if estrogen is the appropriate approach for a specific anxiety patient then I would also prescribe indole-3-carbinol along with it as added protection against estrogen's potential growth stimulation on undetected neoplasms (tumors). I would not use this material in any other circumstances related to the treatment of anxiety.

Take another example. If raising energy seemed useful to augment the anxiety treatment regimen then I might prescribe coenzyme Q10. I might also utilize it if the patient complained of frequent palpitations or heart flutter during panic or intense fear. In each of the following nutrient listings I have indicated the conditions when the nutrient would be appropriate.

5-hydroxytryptophan (5-HTP)

This over-the-counter supplement is a precursor molecule in the synthesis of neurotransmitters that regulate mood and behavior as it effectively increases the central nervous system synthesis of serotonin, the brain neurotransmitter. As discussed previously, serotonin levels have been implicated in depression, anxiety, pain sensation, and sleep regulation. In a study published in the October 1998 issue of *Alternative Medicine Review*, researchers reported that supplementation with 5-hydroxytryptophan has been shown to improve symptoms of depression, anxiety, insomnia, and somatic pains in a variety of patients with fibromyalgia, an arthritis-like syndrome with symptoms of deep muscle pain, anxiety, and depression.

5-HTP is also the precursor for melatonin, which is key to sleep cycles. It has been reported to decrease dopamine and norepinephrine concentrations in the central nervous system, which may influence emotional behavioral processes.

I recommend taking 50 mg of 5-HTP three times a day for generalized anxiety disorder, social phobia, panic disorder, agoraphobia, obsessive-compulsive disorder, and post-traumatic stress disorder. You can increase to 100 mg of 5-HTP three times a day, if needed.

SAM-e

SAM-e (S-adenosyl-methionine), a direct metabolite of the essential amino acid L-methionine, has been prescribed in Europe for pain and depression for more than twenty years. Researchers believe that SAM-e increases the synthesis of neurotransmitters such as serotonin, norepinephrine, and dopamine, all vital for mood regulation. Yet, unlike traditional antidepressants, the mood elevation is felt in the body within days to two weeks (compared to three or four weeks). SAM-e rarely produces the side effects associated with traditional antidepressants such as insomnia, nervousness, nausea, and sexual dysfunction. SAM-e also helps ease anxiety and boost stage 4 sleep.

In a review of evidence from the Agency for Healthcare

Research and Quality, a federal agency aligned with the National Center for Complementary and Alternative Medicine, researchers found that compared to placebo, treatment with SAM-e was associated with an improvement of approximately six points in the score of the Hamilton Rating Scale for Depression measured at three weeks. This degree of improvement is statistically as well as clinically significant.

I recommend taking 400 mg of SAM-e four times a day for any form of anxiety that is worsened by depression. Patients with bipolar disorder should not take SAM-e, as it might cause a manic phase.

Indole-3-carbinol

Indole-3-carbinol is a specific compound that comes from cruciferous vegetables such as cabbage, broccoli, cauliflower, and Brussels sprouts. This nutrient is classified as a sulfur-containing chemical that is a natural antioxidant. It is a potent stimulator of detoxifying enzymes, which makes it a natural deterrent to cancer. I utilize indole-3-carbinol as a cancer deterrent for insurance when a patient elects to utilize estrogen replacement therapy.

I generally recommend taking 200 mg of indole-3-carbinol twice a day when using the hormone estrogen to reduce anxiety. You can get indole-3-carbinol in broccoli, Brussels sprouts, cabbage, cauliflower, collards, kale, kohlrabi, mustard greens, rapeseed, rutabagas, and turnip greens.

Coenzyme Q10 (CoQ10)

Coenzyme Q10 is a fat-soluble, vitamin-like compound that is known as ubiquinone. CoQ10 is also a mandatory nutrient in the tiny energy producers, the mitochondria, present in all cells. As we age, this natural substance is produced in fewer amounts.

I utilize CoQ10 along with two other nutrients, acetyl carnitine and alpha lipoic acid, when I want to strengthen the energy- (mitochondrial-) generating system of the cells, the nerve cells in particular. It is critical that there be efficiency in the energy system of nerve cells in the various parts of the brain that regulate excitement and emotions.

I recommend taking 100 mg of CoQ10 twice a day for patients who suffer fatigue and/or shortness of breath with anxiety.

Alpha Lipoic Acid (ALA)

Alpha lipoic acid (ALA), one of the most potent antioxidants, is both fat- and water-soluble. This vitamin-like nutrient reverses insulin intolerance (as seen with patients who have diabetes and hypoglycemia), which, in turn, reduces hypoglycemia and food sensitivity. Alpha lipoic acid is usually combined with coenzyme Q10 and acetyl carnitine (an amino acid) to improve the energy system in all cells in the body but especially nerve cells in brain areas that control emotions.

I recommend taking 300 mg of alpha lipoic acid three times a day for any anxiety associated with diabetes, hypoglycemia, fatigue, or shortness of breath. Food sources of alpha lipoic acid include organ meats, broccoli, Brussels sprouts, peas, spinach, tomatoes, and rice bran.

Pyridoxal-5-phosphate (P5P)

P5P is the more active form of vitamin B_6, which is critical to the proper functioning of most enzyme systems in the body. I recommend P5P to expedite the conversion of amino acids to neurotransmitters. P5P is also used to alleviate premenstrual anxiety in a fair percentage of women.

I recommend taking 100 mg of P5P once a day when an environmental sensitivity is worsening anxiety.

Methylsulfomethane (MSM)

Methylsulfomethane is a dehydrated form of the solvent frequently used for arthritis called DMSO. I use MSM to help older adults with chronic inflammation get sounder sleep.

I recommend taking 250 to 500 mg of MSM at bedtime for those whose sleep is disturbed by chronic pain and inflammation.

Melatonin

Melatonin is a biochemical with many functions, one of the most important being its well-known relationship with sleep. Melatonin regulates the human biological clock, causing a "phase shift" of the sleep cycle. It may help to raise levels of serotonin, the brain neurotransmitter that influences mood and increases calmness. Some small studies have shown melatonin to improve deep sleep in those with depression. My patients find melatonin especially helpful when high levels of arousal associated with racing thoughts, worrying, or rumination may delay sleep onset, or worries may cause restless sleep and early awakening.

I initially recommend taking a 3 mg capsule of melatonin before bedtime for any anxiety patient who has difficulty falling asleep. If necessary, gradually work up to the dose that provides rest, not to exceed 12 mg of melatonin a day. It may take a few days to get used to this sleep aid, but in most cases, this natural supplement does give benefit.

MAKE A SAFE ASSESSMENT

After reviewing Step 2 as described in this chapter, call your doctor and talk about the benefits and risks of natural therapies to ease anxiety and boost optimal health. A good rule of thumb is to make sure the following two criteria are met:

1. The natural treatment makes you feel better; and
2. The natural treatment does not hurt you in any way.

While it's important to be open-minded about using natural dietary supplements for anxiety disorders, you also need to use your common sense and make sure the supplements you take are safe for your situation.

Chapter 7

Step 3: Eat for Energy

While there are no magic foods that are proven to cure anxiety, research has shown that there are some positive nutritional measures you can take to heal your body. I believe that a healthful diet filled with immune-boosting nutrients can increase energy and alertness, while minimizing the constant fears, anxiety, and fatigue you might feel.

Good solid energy changes the way problems are evaluated in the mind. After all, it is easy to feel emotional, anxious, or depressed when you don't feel good physically. But when feeling strong and healthy, you know you have the energy to think through your problems and shape your future in any way you want. Thus, energy is power. In this case, increased energy provides you with inner power to overcome the bad things that happen to you. The amount of energy you feel determines whether you will project a positive or negative future.

That's why I encourage patients to follow my guidelines in this step and eat to boost energy. In doing so, they lower their anxiety naturally.

Bear in mind that this section is not intended to be a full

discussion of the key parts to a healthy diet. Such information can be found in other books or on the Internet. Rather, I wrote Step 3 with two purposes in mind:

1. To introduce you to some specific nutrients that will increase your energy (the greater your energy, the lower your anxiety and fears); and
2. To help you to stabilize your physical health and mental health with tips on supplementing your daily diet.

We now know that there are distinct connections between the brain, the hormone system, and the immune system. This means that what you eat each day dramatically influences how you think and feel. Following the nutritional suggestions in Step 3 will give you a sense of empowerment.

NUTRITIONAL FACTORS AND ANXIETY

Nutrients are special compounds found in foods that support the body's repair, growth, and wellness. They include vitamins, minerals, amino acids, essential fatty acids, water, and the calorie sources of carbohydrate, protein, and fat. The body makes some nutrients (nonessential nutrients), yet others must come from the diet (essential nutrients). A deficiency of either type of nutrient can lead to illness if left untreated.

I want to focus on some specific nutrients in this section, including carbohydrates, proteins, and essential fats. All three can greatly affect your emotional state and can be manipulated (i.e., eating more or less) to help lessen fears and anxiety while increasing energy and wellness.

Good Carbs, Bad Carbs

Regardless of whether the media blames America's weight problem on diets high in carbohydrates, we still need carbs because they give us a ready source of fuel for energy. In fact, "good" carbs eaten at the right time help get you through the day without feeling anxious and fatigued. The innovative research of Dr. Judith Wurtman of the Massachusetts Institute of Technology reports that selecting certain carbohydrates rather than proteins may actually calm us down, providing almost a self-medicating effect. Conversely, eating "bad" carbs such as pastries loaded with sugar can cause you to feel a sudden burst of energy followed by fatigue, exhaustion, and malaise.

I organize carbohydrates in two categories:

1. Those you should eat moderately ("good" carbs); and
2. Those you should seldom eat ("bad" carbs).

Good or complex carbs include most of your high-fiber fresh fruits and vegetables—from broccoli, cabbage, and bok choy to apples, oranges, limes, and cantaloupes. Because fiber coats the stomach lining, it delays stomach emptying and slows digestion and sugar absorption after a meal, reducing the amount of insulin needed. This insulin response is what can trigger your emotional chemistry, making you feel nervous and anxious or sluggish and fatigued.

However, some complex carbs such as corn, potatoes, rice, soy, and whole grains can also upset your emotional chemistry—just like the simple sugar carbs. Many of my patients are overly sensitive to these carbs, particularly rice and soy. And because these two foods are frequently overused, it makes them more likely to be a hidden source of problems.

What we call the bad carbs include those made with simple sugars such as candy, cakes, pies, pastries, cookies, ice cream, and sweet colas, among others. These carbohydrates cause blood sugar levels to soar and then fall, which triggers your emotional chemistry and results in moodiness or nervousness. Especially for someone with an anxiety disorder, it will be next to impossible to end your symptoms if you load up on bad carbs.

For many of my patients, sugar is one of those foods they can't live with, and they can't live without. However, sugar also is a proven trigger for anxiety and panic in some sensitive people. While carbohydrates are necessary for physical performance and mental energy, you do not need the wrong ones. Here are some suggestions I give to patients on how to incorporate sugar in their diet in a healthy way:

• When eating sugar, always eat a protein food or oil, so the sugar is not flooding your system and overwhelming your glucose-insulin balance. Over time, excessive sugar can cause a breakdown in this balance.

• If you eat many sugar-laden foods, take extra B vitamins because sugar over-utilizes these in the body. Simple sugars or large amounts of high-sugar-content foods trigger a robust metabolic response by our biochemistry. This metabolic surge of activity draws down the B vitamin and mineral reserves needed by the enzymes that process the sugars through our system.

• If you eat a large amount of sugary foods, always add extra potassium supplements (pages 183–184) to your diet to compensate for the over-utilization of potassium by sugar. I find 100 to 200 mg of potassium helpful. Low potassium levels can lead to chronic fatigue, leg cramps, and skin irritation. Likewise, either extremely high or extremely low levels of potassium can be a threat to our heart. (Anyone with a known heart ailment should always check with their doctor before adding or deleting potassium from their diet regardless of whether they are taking medications or not.)

• Sugar causes water retention more than salt in about 95 percent of people. The rule is that 1 ounce of sugar holds in approximately 1 pound of water (about an average cup) for three days. It always amazes me how cardiovascular specialists warn heart and hypertensive patients not to overdo the salt, yet they never mention sugar or alcohol!

Good Carbs, Bad Carbs

Choose Good Carbs

- Low-fat dairy products
- Low-fat protein, tofu, nuts, and legumes
- Nonstarchy vegetables
- Breakfast cereals based on wheat bran, barley, and oats
- Whole grain breads made with whole seeds
- Barley, pasta, and rice instead of white potatoes

Avoid Bad Carbs

- White potatoes
- Refined grains
- Vegetables high in starch such as corn
- Candy
- Pastries

Protein Boosts Alertness

Proteins provide the structural building blocks for growing organs, especially muscles. These foods are associated with increased feelings of alertness, concentration, and performance, as well as sustained energy and balanced moods. Unlike bad carbohydrates, protein foods like turkey, tuna, or chicken are also rich in the amino acid L-tyrosine. L-tyrosine boosts levels of dopamine and norepinephrine, two neurotransmitters (discussed on pages 89–90) that send messages from cell to cell. Research has revealed that people are more alert when the brain is producing these neurotransmitters. When we eat protein food, this increases the amino acid L-tyrosine, which boosts the levels of these key brain chemicals. In turn, we feel alert and can concentrate easier.

Foods high in protein don't trigger the emotional highs and lows of the insulin cycle in the body. When you eat protein, you avoid getting that roller-coaster effect that happens after eating a plate of sugary desserts.

Protein is also important in repairing body tissue and in fighting infection. Too little protein can lead to symptoms of weakness, apathy, and poor immunity.

One ounce of meat, chicken, cheese, or fish provides 7 grams of protein; 1 cup of milk provides 8 grams of protein. Vegetable proteins, such as black beans or tofu, can make a good substitute for animal protein.

As you experiment with the influence of various foods on your emotional state, you'll find that protein will cause an increased alertness for up to two to three hours after the meal—not days or weeks. Likewise, some carbs will help you to stay calm for up to two or three hours after a meal. The effects of food on mood may vary among people and be more intense in some than in others.

Protein Powerhouses

- eggs
- fish
- dairy products
- beef
- poultry
- soy
- legumes

Drink Water to End Fatigue

A few years ago, when some of my patients complained of daytime fatigue, I suggested that they simply drink more water. These same patients later reported that the water did, in fact, boost their energy for a while. Because more than two-thirds of your body weight is water, this liquid is just as important as oxygen for keeping you alive. Imagine every cell, tissue, and organ—all depending on water to function. Water keeps your body alive by stabilizing the temperature, eliminating toxins and waste products, carrying nutrients throughout the body, and maintaining blood volume. You may be surprised to hear that two or more glasses of water, one after the other, is stimulating and can boost energy for thirty minutes to an hour.

Essential Fats

Fats, oils, and lipids (cellular fat content) are as much a part of human nourishment as carbohydrates, proteins, and water. Lack of the proper oils represents malnutrition, equal if not more so, than a vitamin or protein deficiency. Fats, oils, and lipids are also linked to long-term recovery of our emotional and physical health.

Use Oils to Diminish Anxiety?

- Oils are calming.
- Oils boost energy.
- Oils stabilize cell membranes.
- Oils control hormone balance.
- Oils are related to sugar and insulin, which influence emotional stability.

How fats work. Essential fats are classified as omega-3 oils, found in fatty fish, and omega-6 oils (linolenic and gamma-linolenic acid or GLA), found in plants such as evening primrose, black currant, and borage. Some nonessential oils associated with negative effects on the body include omega-9, omega-7, saturated fats, and trans fats.

Our bodies cannot make essential fats, so we must ingest them daily to maintain health. These essential fatty acids (EFAs) have many duties. They regulate inflammation, relax or contract muscles, are turned into tissue hormones (prostaglandins, leukotrienes, thromboxanes), or are incorporated into cell walls. Every cell in your body depends on a proper balance of essential fatty acids for its optimal function.

This includes the brain, nerves, eyes, skin, and blood vessels, among others.

Good fats, bad fats. You would think that the only oils we would ever need would be the unsaturated fatty acids, but that's not so. Unsaturated fatty acids spoil or become rancid rapidly. They are susceptible to free radical activity, discussed on pages 139–140. To keep the food from spoiling before it gets to market, the food industry has resorted to hydrogenating or saturating the fats. Saturated fats are often referred to as trans fats. Trans fats make up some of the material that resides in plastic.

Vegetable fats that are hydrogenated end up looking and smelling like dark grease. They are then bleached, deodorized, flavored, and colored before they are sold as margarine or another form of synthetic fat.

Partially hydrogenating oils is an attempt to walk the line between the best and the worst. Here we get margarine, cookies, snacks, candies, and millions of prepared foods. The starting oils for this conversion come from seed oils, palm, coconut, soy, olive, and peanut oils, among others. The resulting trans fats from this conversion are unfortunately insidiously damaging to metabolic functions as numerous studies have proven. Is that all there is to the story? No! It is really more the type of saturated fat and the amount ingested that becomes the problem.

Saturated fats are not that bad. The saturated fats natural to our diet include butter, coconut and coconut oil, palm kernel oil, and cocoa butter.

Some of the saturated fats are short-chained fatty acids, meaning they are easy to absorb and easy to convert to energy; therefore, a good energy source. Short-chained fatty acids improve the effect of the thyroid hormone because they cause tissues to be more sensitive to it. They can reduce gut mucosal irritation as seen in irritable bowel syndrome and colitis.

A diet too low in saturated fatty acids may cause a hypothyroid-like condition instigating symptoms of fatigue, edema, weight gain, and elevated cholesterol. Excessive amounts of unsaturated fatty acids can become immuno-suppressive, while saturated fatty acids stimulate the immune system and retard the growth of some neoplasms.

Saturated fatty acids are supportive to the kidneys. The kidneys can use saturated fats for a quick energy source if needed.

Unfortunately, there is not much of a correlation between anxiety and saturated fats. Any benefits would be strictly from this effect on energy and thyroid hormone enhancement.

Sugar's negative effect on oils. A diet high in sugar and starch is thought to be behind the development of insulin resistance, which happens when a dietary excess of sugar increases enzyme activity involved in processing fatty acids. This leads to increased production of arachidonic acid. All of this works together to elevate inflammatory conditions such as hypo-glycemia, diabetes, and insulin resistance. As the increased enzyme activity escalates, growing amounts of saturated fats appear in cell membranes. This further complicates insulin resistance. Fish oil supplementation (discussed below) reverses the process, although not rapidly.

Sugar binds into a glycerol group and then attaches to small molecules of fat in the blood to make you fat. When we eat too much sugar for the body to dispose of, the extra sugar snatches up three available fatty acids (fatty acids are always available in the blood) and slips them into our adipose tissue to stow away. Triglycerides are three fatty acids attached to a

sugar group molecule. The body prefers this form of fat because it is perfect for storing.

How to Balance Essential Fatty Acids

· Take a balanced formula of essential fats. The oil
should contain 1 part fish oil or flax oil to 3 parts evening
primrose oil. The quickest and easiest way to arrive at a
balance in your essential fatty acids is to purchase a product that already has that balance. I have listed one in the
Resources called Body Biobalance made by BodyBio. You
can ask for a similar product at your natural food store.

· Include omega-3 fatty acids (alpha-linolenic acid found
in flax seeds and oil, pumpkin seeds, soy beans, walnuts,
and dark green leaves). The marine form of omega-3 fatty
acid comes from cold water fish, including salmon, trout,
mackerel, and sardines, among others. This type of marine oil is referred to as eicosapentanoic acid (EPA) and
docosahexenoic acid (DHA).

· Include omega-6 fatty acids (linolenic acid found in saf-
flower, sunflower, and sesame seeds). Another form, gamma-
linolenic acid (GLA), is found in evening primrose oil.

· I find that 3 servings of cold water fish each week takes
care of the omega-3 requirement in the average person.

· Add a little saturated fat several times each week including butter, coconut and coconut oil, palm kernel oil,
and cocoa butter.

· For further balance, add some omega-9 oils, including
olive, almond, pecan, cashew, and macadamia nut oil. Excessive use of olive oil can cause a buildup of long-chain
fatty acids so now and then use a different oil for a while.

> • Since good mineral balance is a limiting factor in lipid efficiency, it is wise to take an additional mineral supplement such as kelp.
> • It's helpful to use a protein with the oil. Many patients like to mix the oil in cottage cheese.

VITAMINS, MINERALS, AND ENERGY

I discussed many of the key vitamins and minerals I recommend for specific types of anxiety in Step 2 (see Chapter 6). I now want to introduce you to some vitamins that can actually boost energy. I believe that extra energy helps to decrease anxiety—the key is knowing when and how to use the specific vitamin therapies.

I use nutrients as multitasking agents. This may seem strange to some yet interesting to others. The traditional approach is to think of common supplements as preventive-reparative agents, not as drugs. I find many uses for nutrients beyond those that have been assigned by manufacturers or nutritionists.

B Vitamins

I have watched patients experience a great reduction in their feelings of distress after they discontinued their B vitamins. How can a simple vitamin tablet have such a profound effect on the emotional state? While B vitamins help to increase energy, if you take too high a dose, it can result in additional tension and anxiety.

B vitamins are powerful coenzymes to many catalysts in

the body. They have the capacity to jump-start the energy cycle dramatically. Nevertheless, they can also speed it to a steady roar, which is more than enough to make your body and mind shake, rattle, and roll!

Many manufacturers who make multivitamins start with the Bs. When the amount is between 25 and 100 milligrams, most people feel energetic and alert. I like the amount of Bs present to be less than 100 milligrams of each B vitamin to start with.

In my clinic, we have excellent results, including increased energy and lowered anxiety, when we use the combination B vitamins by intramuscular injections. The results are even better when we give the B vitamins in a cocktail mixture of vitamins and minerals, along with other nutrients, all mixed in an IV. In this format, the effects are much more long-acting, especially when the nutrient formula turns out to be a good match to the patient's metabolism.

B vitamins revived Thomas from his burnout. In a recent case, Thomas, a fifty-seven-year-old attorney, came to me having suffered an economic disaster following a precipitous psychological decline. Thomas had built a very successful and growing law practice but wore himself out doing so. In reviewing his medical history, I was convinced he had suffered a physical breakdown before his mental problems. Without warning, he suddenly seemed to fail everywhere, finally falling into total exhaustion. He began having panic attacks and generalized anxiety that culminated in a social phobia. Feeling defeated, Thomas dissolved his firm and became a recluse in a period of a few short months.

Thomas said he came to my clinic because he heard I would avoid if possible prescribing drugs. I immediately started him on my B vitamin injections and within a few days his symptoms markedly declined. You will note I did not opt to start him on tranquilizers or other drugs, which would be a likely scenario had he found a typical physician. The lesson here is that there are alternatives to drugs if doctors wish to administer them.

A key factor in Thomas's medical history that caught my attention was when he said that his anxiety and panic came when he was tired but not when his energy level was high. Unfortunately, a greater part of the time he was fatigued. He also reported he had severe insomnia, which was obviously one of the causes of his fatigue. The traditional physician would have quickly discounted his report of fatigue and insomnia. To me, these symptoms were opportunities to build on.

In addition to the B vitamin injections, I asked Thomas to take some natural remedies for insomnia, including Body Enhancer (see Resources). At this early point in the program, he needed something to ensure quality sleep and something to boost energy. As you would anticipate, my patient's symptoms reduced by about 80 percent. No, I did not prescribe him a sedating, addictive medication. I admit that a drug might have worked just as rapidly and would certainly have been medically indicated. However, Thomas wanted to get well without drugs—and he knew my background and professional experience supported just that.

Help for controlling appetite. Candace, an ER nurse, came to me asking for help with her appetite. This thirty-nine-year-old woman was gaining weight at an alarming rate, but was much too ravenously hungry to halt the disaster that lay ahead, if she didn't stop gorging herself. Candace requested a remedy to block her ravenous appetite. We spent quite a long time reviewing her personal and medical history leading up to the onset of this problem. Then I asked Candace what medications and natural dietary supplements she took. She was on no medications except for an aspirin once in a while, but Candace did say she was taking a high-dose vitamin B complex supplement.

I told Candace that B vitamins are notorious for stimulating appetite when they are at overdose levels. She immediately discontinued the high-dose B vitamins and within two days her appetite returned to normal.

My starting point in discussing B vitamins is that the *right dose* is what we are after—not the highest dose. In fact, I frequently ask patients who are taking B vitamins if their vitamins are pushing them too hard or not hard enough.

Late-life anxiety benefits from B_{12}. Let's look at the link between late-life anxiety and vitamin B_{12}. It is a fact that the mental status of elderly adults sometimes gets as shaky as their bodies. Along with complaints of poor eyesight and arthritis, you can see psychiatric signs and symptoms such as anxiety, depression, agitation, mania, paranoia, delusions, and poor judgment. I've found that some of these symptoms improve considerably with a simple series of vitamin B_{12} injections. Because B_{12} is basically harmless, a single injection is frequently more than enough to determine its value to a person's symptoms. The other benefit to this treatment is that B_{12} boosts energy and that alone is enough to lower anxiety in most people.

If you are planning to use B vitamins for energy, be prepared to work out which brand to use and how much is just right.

Get your Bs naturally. Eat plenty of chicken, fish, liver, kidney, pork, bananas, spinach, sweet potatoes, white potatoes, garbanzo beans, walnuts, brown rice, soybeans, sunflower seeds, avocados, oats, peanuts, lima beans, peanut butter, prunes, and whole wheat products.

Salt

Salt crystals are another natural way to increase your energy immediately. In this regard, I am speaking here of using Celtic Sea Salt, just a crystal or two at a time in water. (Table salt works, too, and you don't have to drive all over looking for it!)

Celtic Sea Salt comes from a seaside area in France (see Resources). This light gray salt retains the full spectrum of ocean minerals. I recommend to patients that they carry a few crystals along with them in a small container or a coin envelope when they are away from home. When they need a pick-me-up energy boost, drop one or two small crystals in a glass of water and drink it. Generally, this will taste only slightly salty and is not objectionable. Almost all of my patients report that it gives them an instant energy and spiritual boost.

I know you are probably getting worried about water retention. But the amount of salt I am suggesting is small compared to the amount one is supposed to ingest daily for good health. I believe that many people have been made phobic of salt by our overly enthusiastic health system, which has lost its perspective. Humans require a minimum of 5 grams or about 1 teaspoon of salt daily or they will become malnourished. If you just can't stop worrying about water retention, I tell my patients to take a tablet or capsule of calcium with the sodium. The reason for this is that the combination of salt and calcium together seems to nullify the water-retaining effects of sodium, a problem women most fear. It is important to note that I did not say one should take calcium daily in the morning or any other time of the day. I said they must be taken together— calcium and sodium together. Together means *at the same time!* Taking the calcium in the morning or evening is not the same as taking it when you are taking the sodium. I don't know why this is such a hard message to get across but it is.

Easing Low Blood Sugar Naturally

Hypoglycemia is a well-known phenomenon to most people. When the blood sugar drops too low, people feel bad but they feel bad in different ways. Some get depressed; some angry; some spacey; and many just become tired and listless. When the blood sugar takes this course, it produces profound effects on many systems. The energy system is obviously affected.

So how do you handle this problem? Most nutritionists suggest eating small snacks throughout the day and not letting too much time go by in between. The snacks should not be sugary because sugar makes the problem worse. Instead, the best advice is to use the salt technique just described.

Another and even better plan, although difficult to follow, is to lightly salt a slice of protein, turkey or chicken for example, and eat it when you feel the beginnings of a hypoglycemic attack. Meat and salt together will provide hours of relief from hypoglycemia and the combination offers a relatively low calorie snack if weight is a problem.

Older nutritionists firmly believe (and so do I) that another word for hypoglycemia is *acidity*. Any supplement that will reduce acidity frequently eliminates symptoms of hypoglycemia. For a list of suggestions, see the section on food sensitivities on pages 189–190.

I advise patients to take 300 mg of alpha lipoic acid (page 163), twice daily, because of its ability to prevent insulin resistance, another cause of hypoglycemia. Be sure to eat food when taking this, or it can upset your stomach.

Potassium

There are many symptoms produced by low tissue potassium levels and one of them is fatigue and inertia. I estimate that I see about 7 to 10 percent of patients who are low in potassium—enough to result in great fatigue. Because blood always takes precedent over tissues, laboratory tests on blood potassium levels often induce erroneous confidence. The blood potassium levels can appear normal when, all the while, the patient is demonstrating signs and symptoms of a potassium deficiency. This deficiency is confirmed when the symptoms disappear after potassium is added, despite the test results.

There is an epidemic of people in this country who have chronic low potassium that seems to result from various causes. It is not so much that our diets are inadequate even though many times they actually are depleted of potassium. Instead, the culprit is frequently that our losses of potassium are greater than our gains.

One of the tip-offs to this problem is fatigue with the additional symptom of inertia (laziness). If the patient tells me they seem to have no motivation in addition to being tired, I begin to search for lifestyle activities that could be depleting their potassium stockpile. A diet high in sugar or alcohol could be the problem because both those items chronically drain off potassium. Natural diuretic teas or medicinal diuretics also will drain off significant amounts of potassium (even if their doctors tell them it won't). Advising people to eat a banana a day is insufficient advice for most people on diuretics, especially if their diet or other compromising factors are unbalanced. Excessive physical activity will over-utilize potassium. Exercise enthusiasts or those participating in heavy physical labor may see chronic deficiencies develop. Large intakes of calcium supplements can reduce potassium levels because the two minerals are in direct competition, one lowering the other if in abundance.

Get potassium naturally. Eat a diet filled with fresh vegetables, cabbage, spinach, bananas, fruit, citrus, and bran flakes.

Calcium

Most of us know we need to ingest calcium, whether in foods or supplements, to keep our bones strong. But did you know that calcium boosts energy in some people, particularly those on weight-loss diets? The idea here is to take the calcium supplementation when your energy is low and not at a set time of the day.

Doctors have known for generations that intravenous calcium will rapidly calm a distraught person. Occasionally, this therapy can backfire and an anxious person becomes extremely agitated. I believe, in the case of these reactive patients, calcium might be lowering, or forcing down, the levels of another mineral, perhaps magnesium, and this causes the paradoxical effect. I have used calcium treatment thousands of times with success, but of late I have replaced it with the glutathione (page 143), which has a more predictable and long-term effect.

Get calcium naturally. Eat plenty of broccoli, bok choy, salmon, sardines with bones, kale, beans (dried), dairy products, soy products, and calcium-fortified foods.

IMMUNE DYSFUNCTION = LOW ENERGY

It has never failed to impress me that when the immune system is suppressed, the feeling of energy is low. How and why these systems are so interrelated is far too complicated to discuss in this book. All I can say from my experience in this area is that when I am successful in raising the patient's resistance, their energy invariably rises. One of the first places to start when faced with this problem is with the adrenal gland. If I feel the immune system is behind the patient's fatigue and the fatigue is contributing significantly to the patient's anxiety, I begin some strengthening procedures. Since there are literally hundreds of immune system enhancers, we have to start somewhere, so here is a typical routine (obviously one routine among many).

Zinc

Zinc has tremendous antioxidant effects and is vital to your body's resistance to infection and for tissue repair. Many illnesses, including kidney disease and long-term infection, are associated with zinc deficiency. If you are taking medication, it may interfere with zinc absorption in the intestines and cause a zinc deficiency. Initially, I recommend 50 to 100 mg to start and may reduce it later. Zinc levels drop like a stone in water when the body is under any sort of physical or mental stress, so the chances are great that this mineral can help you. I don't personally trust hair analysis or most of the other tests to provide an accurate level of a person's zinc, but if you have a physician you trust who does this sort of testing then go with that doctor's program.

Get zinc naturally. Eat plenty of meat, pork, poultry, seafood, wheat products, nuts, seeds, dairy products, and zinc-fortified products.

Colostrum

Colostrum is the first milk made by the breasts for up to seventy-two hours after delivery. It is known to be extremely stimulating to the infant's immune system. Bovine colostrum is commercially available in most health food stores. Some find this to be an excellent immune enhancer. As high-profile as this product is, it still has not risen to the level of becoming a household word. It generally comes in the form of a canister of powder with instructions for proper use. I tell my patients to follow the package instructions.

Probiotics

Probiotics are dietary supplements that contain friendly bacteria. These intestinal microflora are beneficial to the immune system, help you resist infection, and aid in the breakdown of proteins and fats in food, making absorption of vitamins, minerals, and amino acids more efficient. Probiotic bacteria also produce substances called bacteriocins, which act as natural antibiotics to kill unwanted microorganisms.

DR. HUNT'S HOLISTIC RX: EATING FOR ENERGY

The intent of Step 3 is to review the very nutrients that help boost energy and end fears for *all types of anxiety disorders.* After reviewing the summary of recommendations, reread the chapter and mark the specific nutrients that best support your needs.

Start with a Multivitamin

As you eat for energy, start with a broad-spectrum multivitamin that contains minerals and antioxidants. There are many inexpensive ones and it is not necessary to find a super-pill. I usually recommend that patients buy a new brand each time they need a new bottle. They may then find three or four brands that they can rotate. This gives you a greater exposure of nutrients and prevents a continuous metabolic pounding by an individual brand's nutrient formula. Remember, the formulator is making the product for money not because they have some special insight as to the perfect nutrient balance. Nutritional formulas are all totally arbitrary for each nutritional company.

Kelp is an excellent source of minerals and a great addition to a multivitamin. I recommend that at least one bottle be tried along with the multivitamin to see if it adds to the good response.

Add Essential Fatty Acids

Your body does not make essential fatty acids but they are essential for good health. The easiest way to obtain the proper balance is through a product that is already balanced. I recommend a product called Body Biobalance, listed in the Resources. Or you could take at least two capsules of flax oil and four capsules of evening primrose oil daily.

Experiment with Good Carbohydrates and Protein

Work with the good carbohydrates and protein foods listed on pages 170 and 172 to see which foods help calm you down and which foods increase your alertness and productivity. Select calming foods when you are under great stress. Likewise, increase protein foods if you have to be alert.

Ingest Beneficial Bacteria

Eat 1 or 2 servings of yogurt daily. Or take probiotics (acidophilus-bifidus), which are the primary beneficial bacteria found in the gastrointestinal tract. I recommend taking two acidophilus capsules daily.

Avoid Simple Sugars

Avoid simple sugars and any foods that cause a known emotional reaction. Creating insulin chaos by overindulging your sweet tooth is upsetting to your metabolic homeostasis and hard on your emotional stability.

Avoid Food Additives

Avoid environmental sensitivities, especially food additives, if you think you are sensitive to them. Also, avoid tap water unless you are sure the chlorine it contains is not accentuating anxiety.

Drink Plenty of Water

Do drink six to eight glasses of water daily to boost energy levels.

Consider Adding Salt

Make sure you have adequate salt in your diet. Low salt diets cause fatigue and lethargy; tired people have more anxiety. The proper amount is five grams a day. If you are hypoglycemic, make sure you address the problem with simple things like salted protein, salt crystals, salted nuts, and eating frequent small meals.

Eliminate Alcohol

Eliminate alcohol if possible. Alcohol is quick to relieve anxiety but it makes the anxiety worse once it wears off.

Rotate Protein Foods

Many people are sensitive to beef and dairy, so be aware of this possibility. People can become sensitive to chicken also. It is best to rotate all meats and fish, limiting your protein intake to four or five ounces daily. A combination of beans and corn or beans and rice or soy may be used in place of a meat protein if you are not sensitive to corn or rice.

Rotate Grains to Avoid Sensitivities

Grains (wheat, corn, soy, rice, malt, barley, oats) are nutritious foods if you don't have a reaction to them. Try to rotate the types of grain weekly so you don't develop a sensitivity. Most people mistakenly believe that soy and rice are their best friends. I have seen hundreds of patients who are sensitive to these two foods and do not suspect them to be mood-altering.

To check any food for sensitivity, administer the home

neurotoxicity challenge test as described on p. 116. Avoid the food entirely for four days, and then on the fifth day, eat a lot of it. Keep a diary noting any reduction of anxiety during the avoidance period and any reactions upon once again eating it.

Avoid Tropical Fruits

You may be reactive to fruits if there is a pesticide on the skin or if you have a hypoglycemic reaction to the sweetness. In general, tropical fruits such as pineapple and mango are too sugary, so it's best to avoid them. The best fruits are apples, pears, and melons of any type (except watermelon).

Eat Vegetables

Eat unlimited quantities of fresh vegetables except for those most likely to cause hypoglycemia such as potatoes or corn. If cabbage or cabbage juice does not cause you gas, it is calming to an anxious stomach.

Chapter 8

༺ঔৠ

Step 4: Get Calming Sleep

Sleep deprivation was written all over Will's face. While only forty-one, this young attorney looked ten years older with puffy, dark circles under his eyes and a passive blank stare. Will said he went to bed at ten o'clock each night but then tossed and turned until the wee hours of the morning. He always felt too tired to concentrate at the law firm, and his partners were complaining that he seemed distant, distracted, and irritable.

Like Will, many anxiety patients are fatigued and suffer with daytime sleepiness, irritability, and lack of energy. Some patients complain that no matter how long they stay in bed, they just never feel rested. Others get to sleep easily only to awaken frequently throughout the night. Still other patients are convinced that they need little sleep. Lynne, a thirty-six-year-old artist, always got a second wind at night and said she could get the most creative work done after midnight, when her three children were asleep. The problem is that Lynne also had to wake at 6:00 A.M. to dress her children and take them to school. On most mornings, she was exhausted, irritable, and felt high anxiety.

There are so many problems during the day that we tend to

think of sleep as the only real escape. In reality, restlessness and poor-quality sleep due to worries increase the body's anxious state. Problems appear at night when you least expect them. You may experience nightmares, night sweats, night panic, and sudden awakenings because of an excited heart. Muscle twitches, gastric reflux, and hypoglycemic attacks are also common nighttime events. When you add snoring, obstructive sleep apnea, hormone imbalances, and nighttime pain, is it any wonder you have trouble getting a good night's sleep?

In Step 4, I'm going to give you the natural tools to improve your quality of sleep and, in doing so, reduce your anxiety. In my professional opinion, you can reduce your anxiety level up to 50 percent if you simply get a good night's sleep. I emphasize the phrase "good night's sleep" because if you are having trouble sleeping and you manage to get additional sleep, it's still not the same. More sleep or even somewhat better sleep is not good enough; anything short of a solid night's sleep is unacceptable in my clinic.

WHY SLEEP?

We didn't used to have such trouble sleeping at night. More than a century ago, Americans slept an average of ten hours each night. However, that was before the invention of the incandescent lightbulb in 1880. Since Edison's invention, the number of hours Americans sleep has steadily declined. Today, the average American sleeps six and a half hours. Not only can lack of sleep put undue stress on the body, releasing a torrent of stress hormones that increase anxiety, but poor sleep affects overall energy, mood, and productivity.

The topic of sleep has interested researchers for a long time. More than two decades ago, a group of college students participated in a one-month sleep-challenge study. The subjects voluntarily gave up one hour of sleep a night for thirty days. They were tested for a number of psychological factors before the study and then the tests were repeated at the end of the program. In the findings, published in the journal *Medical Educator*, virtually every participant reported one or more personality changes, with symptoms that included impatience, impetuosity, fatigue, irritability, some anxiety and depression, lack of focus, and a number of additional symptoms.

The human body must have a coordinated response to any situation that might disturb its normal function. When daily traumas tear down our homeostatic balance (internal stability), we end our day weaker and more vulnerable to emotional problems and illness. We need relief; and a good night's sleep can set things right again as the circadian rhythms (internal rhythmic twenty-four-hour cycles) are reset, emotional traumas are reprocessed, and memories and thoughts are solidified, among other processes.

The sleep cycle is the control center for a positive state of equilibrium. Without this internal balancing effect, neither the mind nor body will function well. This internal balancing center controls the ultradian rhythm or physiological cycles that occur a number of times within a twenty-four-hour period. Regular fluctuations throughout the day are a hallmark of almost all living organisms. Every physiological event in our body is under the influence of these cycles, so the more normally they function, the better our mental and physical health.

Any attempt on your part to avoid a full night's sleep will fail because the sleep center will persistently make you sleep throughout the following day. With one hour of good sleep, you earn about two hours of energized wakefulness. Nevertheless, let's say you sleep only six hours instead of eight. You've only stored twelve hours of energy that you must now stretch out over an eighteen-hour day. Clearly, you will notice your lack of energy the next day!

THE STAGES OF SLEEP

The purpose of sleep is not to rest. You can rest quietly in bed throughout the night. However, if you don't sleep well, your mind and body will pay a heavy price. During sleep, brain waves constantly change as you pass through the different stages, cycling every ninety minutes from deep to shallow stages. This process is essential to good health and the highest level of functioning.

The five stages of sleep are distinct with specific characteristics defined by brain waves, eye movements, and muscle tension. The two broad categories of sleep include rapid eye movement (REM) sleep and non–rapid eye movement (NREM) sleep.

Rapid Eye Movement Sleep (REM)

The ocular activity with REM sleep is beneficial to the body in a number of ways. First, it is a mechanism the body uses to prevent our awakening. We avoid arousal when the eyes saccade (jump back and forth), allowing us to seamlessly continue back down the cycle into deeper sleep. Secondly, and even more important, rapid eye movement produces imaging or dreaming so that we can process past events.

During REM, we actively rearrange our image/thought/emotional balances, thus stabilizing our new memories. We experience small, variable-speed brain waves, rapid eye movements like those of eyes-open wakefulness, and no muscle tension. We have almost all our dreams during REM sleep. This stage is associated with psychological well-being and we feel refreshed upon awakening. Young adults spend about 25 percent of their sleep time in REM; by age sixty, REM sleep can be as low as 15 to 20 percent of sleep time. If you are deprived of REM sleep, you might complain of increased anxiety, irritability, and moodiness.

Non–Rapid Eye Movement Sleep (NREM)

You go through four different levels in NREM sleep, which are characterized by different combinations of brain waves, eye movements, and reduced but not absent muscle tension. Stages 3 and 4 are important, as they are defined by relatively large, slow brain waves (called delta waves), absent eye movements, and reduced muscle tension. Stage 3 is characterized by extremely slow (delta) brain waves interspersed with very quick brain waves; stage 4 sleep is made up entirely of delta brain waves. Not only does stage 4 sleep allow you to feel alert and energetic and be more productive, it is also vital for restoring your body—repairing tissues and skin, building bone and muscle, and strengthening immune function. Some recent sleep studies show that delta sleep is vital for physical recovery.

Delta sleep, which occurs mostly in the first third of the night, makes up about 10 to 20 percent of total nighttime sleep in normal young adults. This stage is affected by age, amount of prior sleep, various diseases, and physical or emotional trauma. Not surprisingly, young children have large amounts of delta sleep. During delta sleep, human growth hormone (HGH) is abundant, so the rate of tissue repair and cellular growth is at its highest. If sleep disturbances occur during these stages, you will wake up feeling tired and may complain of muscular aches and pains.

Dream Sleep

Although it's possible to dream in any of the four NREM sleep stages, we almost always dream in REM sleep. The dream sleep state takes place during the last third of your night's sleep and normally comprises 35 percent of the sleep period. During the dream sleep state, hormones from the brain stem paralyze the entire skeletal system, presumably to prevent us from hurting ourselves by acting out our dreams as we sleep. Ironically, eye muscles are the exceptions; the eyeballs move about just as if we were awake and active. Experts believe that the function of dream sleep in adults is to reinforce the neural connections between brain cells that are necessary to make memories stick.

Young children have large proportions of delta sleep, which increases if they are sleep-deprived. Elderly adults have smaller proportions of delta sleep, which is why they are easily awakened by environmental noise. Medical problems such as periodic leg movements, obstructive sleep apnea, and pain-related ailments like fibromyalgia can affect quantity and quality of delta sleep.

The Five Types of Sleep

Stage 1—light sleep
Stage 2—moderate sleep
Stages 3 and 4—deep or delta sleep
Stage 5—REM (rapid eye movement) sleep or dream
    stage

Normal and Abnormal Sleep Patterns

Most people go through the five cycles during sleep, ranging from rapid eye movement at the apex of the cycle, then descending all the way down into deep stage 4 sleep at the bottom. Each of these stages is important to normal levels of alertness the following day. If we are deprived of any of these stages of sleep, we will suffer later.

Humans are on a ninety-minute ultradian cycle, causing mental energy to rise and fall, like ocean waves. We barely notice these cycles during our waking hours. Yet during sleep there are more pronounced highs and lows and it is during the crest of each wave that we pass through the rapid eye movement stage. Apparently, this activity provides the brain an opportunity to rearrange its circuitry. Experts believe that the neurological connections linking our sensory visual-imagery experiences (sight, sound, touch, and taste) of traumatizing events are weakened or completely disconnected by REM sleep. The purpose of this processing phase is to reduce the previous day's stress by readjusting the emotional power connected to prior memories, especially traumatic ones. The next day, if we have had a terrific night's sleep, we notice that we are much less concerned about the previous day's upsets.

When the neurological link between memory and the specific brain area for emotions is weak or nonexistent, then little negativity is felt when we recall a disturbing event. Sleep allows us to cease experiencing life long enough to readjust our cognitive understanding of what is real and what is not. Our emotional stability depends on our not reliving prior stress repeatedly and becoming distressed by our memories. If the brain did not have this capacity to diminish our negative feelings each night, we would be forever accumulating intense, overwhelming emotions. This banking-up of worries would paralyze us. Instead, by sleeping well, we detoxify our emotions through rapid eye movements so that past stresses drop to a controllable level and we are able to focus on the present rather than the past.

Common Sleep Stressors

- Physical symptoms stemming from stress (increased heart rate, anxiety, gastrointestinal problems, difficulty breathing)
- Feeling overwhelmed
- Anxiety upon awakening
- Impatience for no apparent reason
- Inability to sleep soundly
- Difficulty in concentrating
- Loss of interest or enjoyment in life
- Frequent irritability or anger
- Mood swings
- Changes in appetite (eating more or less food)

HOW SLEEP PROCESSES MEMORIES

The current belief is that the front or logical-thinking part of the brain is deactivated during normal sleep. Electrical delta waves during sleep block conscious thinking. It is during this sleep phase when we're unencumbered by mental activity that restorative processes take place (called homeostatic rebalancing). This is also when we solidify our memory. When the quality of the normal electrical rhythms of sleep is poor, there is a dramatic decline in working memory.

A working memory or short-term memory keeps current factors in mind so we can problem-solve. This working memory is critical to making a plan and following through and its efficiency can be effectively measured. Virtually all students with poor grades have poor working memories. Those people who seem to continually fail in life usually test deficient in this area. If you want to improve your working memory, be sure you are passing through all phases of a normal sleep cycle.

This blocking effect on thinking during REM sleep is not continuous. In healthy animals, circuits that are activated during wakefulness are reactivated during REM sleep. It's as though the body is fast-forwarding memories as it stores them, thus bringing closure to the episode. In addition, the emotional (limbic) system in the brain is active during REM sleep as well; that is why we dream. The dream is not logical though, because memories are being shuffled out of sequence, along with past memories that may arise. In schizophrenic patients, where there is a failure to experience adequate REM sleep, memories are kept in the consciousness intact, day and night, where they produce hallucinations.

Normal sleep is important for long-term memory consolidation also; just one more reason why skimping on sleep is a dangerous practice.

Consider a Sleep Study

If your doctor suspects that you might have a sleep disorder, you might be referred for a sleep study called a polysomnography. The sleep study will help determine if you have snoring, obstructive sleep apnea, restless legs syndrome, or other problems. All of these disorders require specific therapy your doctor will prescribe.

THE BENEFITS OF GOOD SLEEP

Sleep is one of the mechanisms the body uses to maintain hormonal balance, which is necessary for emotional stability. If, for example, the energy-charging adrenal glands are denied the benefits of sleep each day, they won't function well enough to do their job. When gender-specific hormones such as estrogen, progesterone, and testosterone get out of balance, you might feel restless and find it hard to relax.

Better Coping Skills

Good sleep increases your coping skills, helping you to manage life's stressors in a healthy manner. Yet more than 50 percent of Americans suffer from fragmentary sleep. If emotional cleansing during REM stage sleep does not occur because of poor or fragmented sleep, then negative emotions pile up and begin to color your thoughts during the day. Every stress becomes more pronounced because it is compounded by past emotional baggage.

Normal people sleep with an efficiency level between 90 and 100 percent. The closer we get to 100 percent, the better. By efficiency, I mean passing completely through all phases of an appropriate number of sleep cycles, and allowing enough time for each phase to fulfill its function. Those who suffer fragmentary sleep have a much poorer efficiency level, and many drop below 50 percent. Findings reported at the seventeenth annual meeting of the Associated Professional Sleep Societies revealed that good sleepers tend to use task-oriented coping skills while poor sleepers rely more on emotionally oriented strategies. That means that the latter are far more emotional and less rational when problems have to be faced. This type of person tends not to make good decisions.

More Energy

A patient of mine once remarked that the natural sleeping aid I gave him was providing him with the best energy of his entire life. I explained to him that the nutrient used was not a stimulant and had no innate ability to energize him. His energy was released naturally, simply a result of his high-quality sleep.

No one needs to garner energy more than someone who is suffering from narcolepsy, a condition where you find it difficult to stay awake during the day and can fall fast asleep at any moment, even while driving. Until recently, physicians were on the right track prescribing amphetamine-class drugs for these patients, who usually require intense stimulation. Often it takes two or three different medications to do the job, and even then, many patients complain about poor results.

Here's where sodium oxybate, also known as gammahydroxybutyrate (GHB), can be put to good use. This supplement increases deep, slow-wave sleep and, in one sense, forces the body through a good night's sleep. The result is no narcolepsy. By restoring the narcoleptic's sleep efficiency, normal energy metabolism is set up for the next day. If anything can prove that a good night's sleep produces energy, this has to be a classic example.

Although legal, sodium oxybate therapy is not generally available, even though the studies show it is a viable solution. A review of studies on sodium oxybate was published in the August 2003 issue of the journal *Current Psychiatry*, concluding that this drug worked well with few side effects. In one study of 136 patients, one participant dropped out because of confusion and nine others had mild but bothersome problems. Twelve patients developed bed-wetting, which stopped when they were advised to urinate before retiring. Sleepwalking was the only major side effect, but all participants in the study managed to live with this by taking proper precautions.

I broach this subject only so you can appreciate why I place so much emphasis on sleep as a source of energy. (Physicians interested in prescribing this medication should check out the reference in the Resources section. The *Current Psychiatry* article contains the phone number where a doctor can order the appropriate forms.)

GOOD SLEEP, BAD SLEEP . . . NO SLEEP

Some people try to avoid sleep by taking stimulants to stay awake. When you combine lack of sleep with long-term use of addictive or pseudo-addictive stimulants that often cause permanent neurotoxicity, then you increase your risk of future health problems. You may get away with taking stimulants for a while, especially if you are young. However, it's unlikely you'll escape damage if you continue to subvert your primary rebalancing mechanism. When you deny yourself sleep, you demonstrate a lack of respect for your body, because you're deliberately undermining its normal functions.

In a study published in a 2001 issue of the German journal *Fortschr Medical Origins*, researchers concluded that one out of four patients suffered from significant insomnia and 75 percent of those questioned had some level of sleep disturbance. Despite the fact that the patients recognized they had a problem, barely 25 percent were taking any action. Physicians were also found to be nonchalant about the seriousness of sleep deprivation and frequently offered no treatment; they just ignored it.

Myriad scientific studies have revealed new insights into the importance of good sleep and the long-term effects of bad sleep or no sleep:

• People with chronic sleep deprivation, sleep disruptions, and daytime sleepiness are more likely to need increased health care for problems such as hypertension, chronic bronchitis, and asthma compared to those with better sleeping habits.

• There is a proven relationship between difficulty falling asleep and coronary artery disease in males.

• Unresolved sleep problems can significantly impede daytime activities.

• Insomnia is a definite risk factor for psychiatric, as well as medical problems, and this is especially true in the case of depression.

• Sleep dysfunctions that result in daytime sleepiness will result in an increase in occupational accidents.

We're also aware that daytime sleepiness may be a sign of early dementia. People who do not sleep well, especially older persons, are usually sleepy the following day. So when we see or hear that someone is drowsy, we assume he has not had a good night's sleep. However, daytime sleepiness does not automatically indicate a problem with nocturnal sleep patterns. In a study reported in the December 2001 issue of the *Journal of the American Geriatric Society*, researchers found that if a person complaining of daytime sleepiness is older, this symptom may be one of the first signs of dementia. If you or someone you know has this problem, talk to your doctor.

RESOLVING SLEEP PROBLEMS

Improved sleep is not relevant in every case of anxiety, but it *is* a key risk factor in a large percentage of cases—no matter what type of anxiety disorder is present. Since half of the general population suffers with chronic sleep problems, it is not surprising that the majority of those with anxiety also have this disorder.

When patients come in for a consultation, I encourage them to describe their sleep habits. I know that if sleep is a problem, a quick intervention in that area will produce a big— and immediate—payoff. A restful night's sleep always lowers anxiety levels. In some cases, quality sleep results in resolving anxiety completely.

Selenium and Nighttime Anxiety

To relieve nighttime anxiety, I use antioxidants very successfully. A good example is using the antioxidant selenium near bedtime to remove the hyperactivity that interferes with the desire to go to bed. Night owls are often those who build up oxygen debt, which generates feelings similar to agitation. These nocturnal people grow more awake as the night goes on even though they have been active all day and ordinarily should be tired and ready for bed. Under these conditions, when they take an antioxidant they tend to feel very sleepy.

End External Environmental Disturbances

While some people can sleep next to a passing train, most of us need peace and quiet when we go to bed at night. Establishing sleep hygiene is important to managing the symptoms of anxiety. Here are some suggestions to control environmental disturbances:

• Don't play the television, radio, or any form of music while you sleep. Stimulus disturbs natural sleep patterns. Foster good sleep habits in your children by preventing them from taking a Walkman or other electronic toys to bed with them.

• Make sure your bedroom is soundproofed, or wear earplugs, if you are bothered by noises during sleep. (Some people prefer white noise—a humming sound produced by a machine.)

• Keep your bedroom dark, well ventilated, and cool. Use a night mask to block light and other distractions.

Beware of Drugs That Can Cause Insomnia

· blood pressure medications
· hormones
· bronchodilators
· nicotine
· decongestants
· over-the-counter pain relievers that contain caffeine

Resolve Internal Environmental Disturbances

There are many internal disturbances that can lead to poor sleep. In most cases, these are easily resolved with natural therapies. Review the common sleep problems below, and then consider the suggested remedy for resolving them.

Middle-of-the-night urination (nocturia). If you are like millions of other adults, you might be getting up one to four times a night to urinate. Even if you get back to sleep easily, it still breaks up the continuity and quality of your sleep.

The best remedy for nocturia is deeper sleep. I assure my patients that I've helped hundreds of people deepen their sleep to a point where they don't awaken all night long (none have wet the bed). In fact, most of the time, the problem is not a full bladder, but rather the fact that one is sleeping so superficially that the slightest internal stimulation is enough to disturb you.

A large number of middle-aged and older male patients tell me they experience middle-of-the-night urinary urgency, sometimes two or three times a night. Virtually every one of them believes that this is a symptom of an enlarged or inflamed prostate. Sure, there's a natural tendency to blame nighttime urinary urgency on the prostate gland, and sometimes it's the cause, but not always. In many instances, the cause is simply less sound sleep due to normal aging. In younger years, the normal buildup of bladder pressure is insufficient to awaken a person. However, as we age, urinary pressure is stimulating enough to awaken us from a lighter sleep. When my patients are able to deepen their sleep, they find that their nightly trips to the bathroom cease.

Nocturnal cystitis. Interstitial (or nocturnal) cystitis is another culprit that can get you up one or more times a night to go to the bathroom. I'm not speaking of a bladder infection or a prostate problem. This condition is much more subtle and difficult to diagnose, even for trained physicians. Two symptoms that might tip you off are pelvic pain and an overactive bladder. Although this disorder is not usually triggered by recurrent bladder infections, it may become the cause of them. Urine tests often show up as normal, so these don't always help.

Part of the problem of interstitial cystitis is that nerves extending from the bladder to the spinal cord become overly sensitive with the impulses bouncing back and forth in a self-perpetuating dance. If you suspect you have this problem, you will need to see a physician for treatment, because self-help won't work here.

Hypoglycemia. Another common cause of nighttime awakening is hypoglycemia or low blood sugar. Hypoglycemics fall asleep easily but wake up again one to three hours after bedtime and have trouble getting back to sleep. The antidote is simple. Have some protein at bedtime. I encourage my patients to eat a lightly salted slice of chicken or turkey before going to bed. The salt is important because it's a major (and overlooked) hypoglycemic control agent. While salt by itself can reverse hypoglycemia, the effects won't last long without the protein. The worst thing a hypoglycemic can do is to eat something sweet near bedtime.

Nocturnal pain. I am particularly sensitive to the fact that older people tend to have chronically inflamed tissues, which are subclinical (felt below the level of awareness) even though the inflammation may not be obvious. Chronic inflammation is considered the result of the normal aging process, and it is a factor that accelerates aging. Older people often report discomfort if they stay in one position too long. This need to change positions contributes to nocturnal restlessness and fragmented sleep. People with fibromyalgia, an arthritis-like syndrome that affects millions, mostly women, also have difficulty sleeping because of deep muscle pain and aching. Anxiety and depression go along with fibromyalgia syndrome.

As a rule, I explore reasons why a patient experiences tenderness in muscles or joints. If I believe that a patient is affected with a subclinical inflammation, I will prescribe a natural anti-inflammatory at bedtime.

The natural anti-inflammatory that I recommend most to my patients is methylsulfonomethane (MSM). This form of DMSO has long been used for the pain of arthritis and has a mild tranquilizing effect. There are virtually no side effects unless you are allergic to sulfur and even then, most people can tolerate it. I tell patients to take between 100 and 500 mg at bedtime if they have any joint or muscle discomfort.

A substitute for MSM is glucosamine sulfate, a natural over-the-counter dietary supplement. In the body, glucosamine is a naturally occurring amino sugar found in human joints and connective tissues. The body uses it for cartilage development and repair. The natural supplement comes from crab shells and can be found at most natural food stores. I suggest 250 to 500 mg of glucosamine at bedtime. (Both of these products may be found in a drink called Body Enhancer described in Resources.)

Imbalanced hormones. Women are trickier to study because of the effects of estrogen on their sleep patterns. Studies show that women have more awakenings, sleep disturbances, and vivid dreams during the premenstrual time than the rest of the month. Some women report having fatigue, no matter how long they stay in bed. Menstrual symptoms such as bloating, headache, abdominal cramps, food cravings, irritability, and emotional changes all contribute to the inability to get sound sleep. These problems generally disappear a few days after menstruation begins.

For women in perimenopause (just prior to menopause), the declining levels of the hormone estradiol may increase their chance of poor sleep. In a study published in the September 2001 issue of the journal *Obstetrics and Gynecology*, researchers at the University of Pennsylvania Medical Center in Philadelphia followed 436 women age thirty-five to forty-nine over a two-year period. About 17 percent of the women reported suffering from poor sleep throughout the entire study period. While researchers blamed anxiety, depression, and caffeine consumption as factors that disturbed the women's sleep, they also identified low estradiol levels and hot flashes in older women aged forty-five to forty-nine as responsible for the sleepless nights, even though the women were experiencing regular menstrual cycles and had not yet entered menopause. The study concluded that the decline in estradiol that occurs with ovarian aging may, in fact, be associated with poor sleep in women. This sleep deprivation results in daytime fatigue and irritability and can even lead to feelings of anxiety and depression.

SAY GOODBYE TO PANICKY NIGHTS

Panicky nights caused by nightmares, night terrors, and other problems can result in daytime sleepiness and higher anxiety. Once you recognize the problem, there are natural therapies you can use to manage it.

Nighttime Trauma

A nightmare is usually a complete dream that is frightening throughout. Or a nightmare leads up to something so horrible that you awaken in a panic. Most nightmares involve some sort of a chase or a sense of being controlled by another person in a rapidly escalating and harmful way. The most prominent symptom is the pervasive feeling of helplessness. The nightmare often occurs near the end of a sleep period. Even if you go back to sleep, you usually will recall the dream the following morning.

While occasional nightmares are universal, about 5 to 10 percent of the population have them frequently. Nightmares occur frequently in younger children, age three to eight. It is thought that as many men have the problem as do women but since men seldom seek help for the problem, the numbers collected are not considered accurate. In my experience women are probably more vulnerable to this problem because of the destabilizing effect of the menstrual cycle. Older people should not consider themselves safe from it even if they have not had any severe ones to date; nightmares can come at any age.

Nightmares are triggered by hormone imbalances and occur frequently with PMS (premenstrual syndrome). Those who suffer with panic attacks, high levels of anxiety, or depression may experience nightmares.

Certain drugs can cause nightmares; among these are beta-blockers, L-dopa, anesthetics, and street drugs. Yet withdrawing from drugs is also a known trigger of nightmares. Stresses such as losing your job, loss of a loved one, divorce, or other major life change are also triggers of nightmares.

Night terror. In contrast to a nightmare, if you have a night terror, you do not remember the experience. Those who undergo night terrors usually signal their ordeal by loudly emitting a terrorized scream, but they frequently do not awaken after doing so. The few who remember anything the following day merely recall sensations of suffocation or pressure on the chest. If an observer attempts to awaken someone in the middle of a night terror, he will find it extremely difficult because night terror patients are groggy and difficult to rouse. Night terrors usually occur early in the night, often not long after you have fallen asleep.

Night terrors are not dreams; they are startling sensations. Body movements that accompany the scream can be sleepwalking. Night terrors have been induced in children by quickly pulling them upright while asleep. Night terrors have been created in post-traumatic nightmare patients (described below) in the same manner. Because it is possible to induce a startle reaction in these individuals, the two disorders very likely are related. Night terror patients, not remembering their nocturnal experience, usually discover the problem when another person tells them. Post-traumatic nightmare patients usually do recall their dreams. There are even people who suffer both nightmares and night terrors.

Post-traumatic nightmare. Post-traumatic nightmares occur, supposedly, as a consequence of some frightening event. This type of bad dream seems to be a cross between a nightmare and a night terror. Biochemically, the dream is closer to a night terror. You experience the terrible event as a dream, but you can remember this later on. You also might sit up and scream with terror or even sleepwalk. Post-traumatic nightmares are fairly common and can occur at any age.

My Personal Experience

When I had surgery about thirty years ago, I was given the anesthetic Ketamine. One of the side effects of Ketamine is lingering nightmares. As I awoke from the anesthetic, I seemed to be coming out of a nightmare in which I was a motionless steel robot, frozen in space and unable to breathe or speak. My inability to breathe and the utter helplessness of my locked-in-position metal limbs caused me great panic.

I eventually came out of it into complete consciousness, but the lingering drug left me with a very unsettled feeling that held on for days. I began reexperiencing this event night after night for a while and then it gradually tapered off into several times a month. It dogged me for two years.

I don't think anyone who suffers with nightmares or night terrors takes it lightly. I dreaded going to sleep and was terribly relieved when the dream finally left. Obviously, this experience was before I was involved in anxiety and nutritional medicine. If I had the same problem today, I would simply take my nutrients. Still, I learned a lot about what those who suffer with panic feel.

Ending Panicky Nights Naturally

To end nightmares and night terrors, I recommend that patients take between 100 and 500 mg of thiamine at bedtime. In most cases, the nightmares disappear immediately. I also have clients search their diet and daily habits for ways thiamine could be depleted. For example, there are certain nutrients like silica that deplete thiamine. Alcohol, sugar, and street drugs also deplete thiamine. Anesthetics also knock out large amounts of B vitamins, including B_1 (thiamine).

Sleepwalking

Although nightmares are uncomfortable, they are not dangerous like sleepwalking, where the result can be injury or even death. In a study published in a 1986 issue of the journal *Psychosomatics,* two scientists studied a young man who fell asleep and woke up several hours later standing in front of his door bleeding from a head injury. Apparently, he had been walking in his sleep and had managed to fall out of his second-story window down twenty feet into some bushes. In the same report another patient wakened to find blood spurting from his wrist; he was jammed halfway through a broken sliding-glass door.

Complex behavior in addition to simple sleepwalking can also occur during these episodes. A case in point is that of a young man who would strike out at people or smash furniture during violent episodes while sleepwalking. In these instances, he was not only a threat to himself but to others as well. His wife was brutally battered during one such event. Another serious case of sleepwalking involved a fifty-year-old man who, feeling tired, pulled his car into a highway rest area for a nap. An hour later, he sat up and started his car but there was one serious problem: He was still fast asleep. He drove his car back onto the highway in the wrong direction. Oncoming drivers swerved, blew their horns and shouted. Zombie-like, staring straight ahead, he roared on through the night. Three people died when he hit their car dead-center.

Keep in mind, there are some known triggers that can precipitate sleepwalking. Most noticeable among the triggers is alcohol. The man above who fell out his window was a heavy beer drinker. The man who walked through the glass door drank excessively on weekends. The man who had the traffic accident had consumed five or six cocktails prior to the drive.

Night Twitches

If you are wondering what I am talking about when I say night twitches, then you probably don't have them. A twitch is a sudden contraction of a muscle group resulting in a small jerk in the body or some part of the body, most often the head or a shoulder. Anyone who shares a bed with a twitcher knows what I am talking about because the bed moves a little with every jerk. Many people have little muscle jerks now and then but the night twitches I am speaking of are definitely rhythmic, usually occurring every five to fifteen seconds.

It is not unusual for a night twitcher to be seen doing it during the day, too. This affliction usually runs in families. A mother and daughter may be twitching at the same time. Twitchers, however, are not always twitching; days may go by between spells. They usually begin doing it after stress and often after eating or drinking something they are sensitive to; sugar or spicy foods are two common triggers. In my experience, there is usually an identifiable trigger that sets off the episode.

Twitchers are seldom aware they are doing it, so the outside observer must be the one to tip them off. A nocturnal twitcher will often change positions while sleeping but not be awakened by the movement. It takes an outside observer to mention it.

The majority of the time, the twitches can be terminated within a few minutes after taking 4 or more mg of the trace mineral manganese prior to bedtime or even during the night. This mineral works most of the time to resolve twitches, but there may be the need to add 800 IU of vitamin E. On several occasions, I have resorted to 250 to 500 mg of the amino acid acetyl carnitine taken at bedtime. All these nutrients may be used for daytime twitching as well. If you or a loved one suffers with twitching, you may want to check with a neurologist for a complete diagnosis.

Nocturnal Acidity

Nocturnal panic is usually caused by a buildup in acidity between the hour of sleep and the time of the attack. If the person has gotten excessively warm or overheated from too many covers or elevated heat in the room, the higher temperature seems to intensify and accelerate the buildup. Another reason for increased acidity is hypoglycemia. While the buildup of an acid state triggers migraines in some people, it causes panic attacks in others.

Eating something at bedtime easily controls hypoglycemia, and I don't mean eating ice cream. Sugars are the perfect food to create acidity. Sugars themselves are acid. They burn off all the vitamins and minerals that buffer against acidity and then they generate hypoglycemia, which is a state of acidity. If anything creates body acidity, it's sugar. I was about to say that the worst thing you can do is have a sweet snack near bedtime but that would be wrong; the worst snack of all is alcohol.

Fruit is pure sugar, so it is just slightly better than table sugar. Fruit is definitely not a bedtime snack for people who could experience a nightmare. Instead, a slice of turkey lightly salted or buttered would be excellent. A bowl of salted nuts is not so bad either as a bedtime snack. The rule of thumb I tell my patients is this:

- Sugar postpones hypoglycemia for 1 hour.
- Protein postpones hypoglycemia for 2 to 3 hours.
- Oils hold off hypoglycemia for more than 3 hours.
- Proteins and oils together outlast any single food, and when you postpone hypoglycemia, you postpone acidity.

Sometimes the symptom that awakens you is not a total panic attack but rather a fast heartbeat and a good deal of worry—not a true panic attack, but a good copy of a panic attack in a milder form.

Nutritional Sleep Aids

Tryptophan, an amino acid, is a precursor in the synthesis of serotonin, a neurotransmitter in the brain associated with a calming, anxiety-reducing reaction. Since tryptophan is present in milk—and warm milk seems to help individuals fall asleep—this amino acid became popular as a home remedy for insomnia and was available as an over-the-counter natural dietary supplement until just a few years ago. For many years, it was *the* reliable natural sleeping aid before the natural hormone melatonin became available (pages 164–165). However, some patients who ingested tryptophan as a dietary supplement developed a syndrome with features of a disease called scleroderma, which included skin tightening, pain in the joints, muscle aches, and weakness. These patients also developed anxiety, depression, and difficulty learning. Some patients actually died. It was later thought that the deaths were due to a contaminant of tryptophan in the substance they took. The Food and Drug Administration removed tryptophan from the consumer market after a single contaminated batch made headlines. You can now get this amino acid by prescription only.

It has been well documented that tryptophan can produce superior sleep efficiency. A dose of 500 to 1,000 mg at bedtime produces a long and powerful sleep. A few people report drowsiness upon awakening, but lowering the dose usually solves the problem.

Most health food stores stock a nutritional product called 5-hydroxytryptophan (5-HTP), which is a derivative of the amino acid tryptophan and boosts serotonin in the body. While 5-HTP may have taken tryptophan's place on the store shelves, it does not have the same power. I've had patients try both and universally they say tryptophan is stronger. Some people like 5-HTP, while others tell me it makes them feel funny or not themselves. I let patients find out for themselves, but I don't prescribe it regularly because of the inconsistent responses.

Magnesium

I discussed the impact of magnesium on emotional health in Step 2 (pages 137–138). This key mineral also plays a key role in regulating both the sleep cycle and the endocrine system. In a revealing study reported in the July 2002 issue of the journal *Pharmacopsychiatry*, researchers studied twelve elderly patients using the sleep electroencephalogram (EEG) and nocturnal hormone secretion. They found that magnesium supplementation led to increased slow-wave sleep during the night.

In this particular study, researchers concluded that while sleep patterns change with aging, magnesium reverses this change, bringing the pattern in line with that of a younger person. Interestingly, the effects of magnesium mimicked the effects of another mineral, lithium, which is used to treat depression and bipolar disorder. This suggests that magnesium may affect a person's mood much in the same way that lithium does.

I find that 100 mg of magnesium taken at bedtime is usually sufficient. Too much magnesium near bedtime acts as a stimulant and can keep you awake. Many times a little goes a long way with natural dietary supplements. In addition, as stated previously, magnesium often works better when combined with other minerals such as calcium.

HORMONES FOR SLEEP

Progesterone

Studies show that the hormone progesterone is rapidly converted into neuroactive steroids that have positive effects on sleep. Progesterone reduces locomotor activity, which is conducive to sleep, and also produces a benzodiazepine-like (tranquilizing) sleep EEG profile, which provides additional aid.

I recommend natural progesterone made from a plant source primarily to men, especially if they snore at night or have mild to moderate sleep apnea, which causes brief periods of breathing cessation during sleep. While not for everyone, 100 to 200 mg of bioidentical progesterone at bedtime can deepen your sleep and make you feel more energized during the day. This product is available only by prescription, although many health food stores sell very weak natural products that slightly mimic the pharmaceutical grade. Progestins will not substitute.

Estrogen

When estrogen starts to decline during menopause, hot flashes come and go responding to the uncontrolled, fluctuating blood calcium levels, and make it difficult to stay asleep. Estrogen is a major moderator of the essential mineral calcium, and calcium is vital in maintaining vascular tone as well as constriction of blood vessels. Hot flashes are caused by dilated blood vessels. Taking one-half teaspoon of liquid calcium during a hot flash can actually terminate the flash. This cannot be recommended on a steady basis because of the possibility of overdosing on calcium, but it could be used occasionally.

Another way estrogen improves sleep is that estrogen reduces excitement in our cerebral alerting system, which is stimulated during REM sleep (when we dream). Some younger people and many older people are awakened by dreams because of the neurological excitement that occurs during that sleep state. Estrogen, in normal amounts, mutes this excitement sufficiently to prevent awakening.

Estrogen does not cause cancer but it is a growth factor and therefore can stimulate abnormal cellular reproduction, thus making it a possible hazard, especially to older and more vulnerable individuals (those with a family history of cancer or past history of breast lumps, cysts, and soreness). Women should never try to circumvent professional care by taking soy products that may contain estrogen to raise their estrogen level on their own. Professional consultations are mandatory where synthetic estrogen or natural forms of estrogen are concerned.

Thyroid

Prescriptive thyroid is a great sleeping aid for some individuals. I ask my hypothyroid patients, to whom I have given a prescription, to try taking their thyroid medication at bedtime if they do not notice it generating excessive daytime energy. In a fair number of cases, they can tolerate it at bedtime and experience a solid night's sleep.

Melatonin

Some patients benefit from the over-the-counter supplement melatonin. In the body, this hormone is produced only at night by the pineal gland in the brain. With sunlight, the body's primary timekeeper, this natural hormone helps to set the brain's biological clock. This clock determines all of the body's circadian rhythms, from hormone releases and body temperatures to the sleep-wake cycle and digestive functions.

In some sleep research studies, scientists report that taking melatonin an hour before bedtime may induce sleep more quickly and continue longer than with a placebo. Most of my patients know melatonin helps with sleep, and they've been told that the proper dose is usually around 3 mg at bedtime. However, the majority of those who have tried it have not found it helpful.

What many people do not know, however, is that there are ways of generating your own melatonin, and these methods can be effective. You can release melatonin in the evening prior to sleep by lowering the level of illumination. The lights from a television are enough to retard the release of melatonin. Reading in bed can be a problem, too.

Normal levels of melatonin are very low during the day and begin to rise around 11:00 P.M., peak around 2:00 to 3:00 A.M., and then begin to drop somewhere between 3:00 and 4:00 in the morning. If you are exposed to light during this decline while sleeping, it can accelerate it. In fact, a single minute of light is enough to eliminate most of your circulating melatonin. I recommend that you place a yellow or red light in the bathroom if you use it in the middle of the night. You can use red or yellow covers on clocks and other lights in the bedroom.

Melatonin is also released when the temperature is lowered, so don't overheat the room. A good trick is to take a hot bath and then dress only in something very light so that you cool off rapidly. Rapid lowering of temperature will help release natural melatonin. Also, it is important to go to bed by 11:00 P.M. or earlier, so you can take advantage of this hormone's natural release cycle.

You will not want to take alcohol or stimulants such as coffee or caffeinated soft drinks close to bedtime. Even very stimulating conversations can excite your nervous system and that will release adrenaline into your blood and completely block melatonin release.

As mentioned, when taking melatonin for sleep problems, most people start with 3 mg. If this dose fails to work, they usually give up and begin searching for something else. However, melatonin is safe at much higher doses. If there are no side effects, I tell my patients to continue increasing the dose each night until they find an amount that works. Most of my patients end up taking between 9 and 12 mg of melatonin at bedtime for good sleep. I tell them that they can also take another 3 to 6 mg during the night, if it's not too near morning. If the second dose produces grogginess on awakening, then we move on to another agent.

Melatonin is usually available in 1-, 3-, and 5-mg capsules as well as 2- and 3-mg extended-release capsules. Tablets are manufactured in approximately the same doses. There also is a 3-mg lozenge and a liquid dropper unit available.

This natural supplement is one of, if not *the* strongest antioxidant known, even more powerful than vitamin E or glutathione. Melatonin decreases cortisol, the body's main stress hormone, which rises as your body fights an overwhelming sense of fatigue. And just as with chronic stress, increased cortisol ages your body, inhibits production of white blood cells (lymphocytes), and compromises your immune system.

Melatonin has been found useful in reducing nocturnal hypertension (high blood pressure), and boosts the immune system by activating T-cells, which protect the body from germs such as viruses, bacteria, parasites, and fungi. Melatonin amplifies any medication used to treat mental disorders. Thus, it's important to consult your doctor before taking this supplement.

Because a single nutrient (or drug) is often insufficient for all of the chemical imbalances, I add other natural substances to strengthen the effects. Two very effective aids are the herbs valerian and/or passionflower. Another item of value is 5-HTP.

As you age, melatonin production declines, and that may be one of the causes of poorer sleep patterns in older adults. The good news is that melatonin stimulates the release of human growth hormone (HGH), a hormone secreted by the pituitary gland in the brain, which has an anti-aging effect.

Other Natural Sleep Therapies

In my experience, some of the more recognized therapies such as hypnosis and biofeedback are far less effective than nutritional therapies. Hypnosis is an artificially induced trancelike state that resembles sleepwalking. The subject is in a highly suggestible state and susceptible to instructions given by the therapist. Biofeedback is based on the idea that when people are given information about their body's internal processes, they can use this information to control the processes. Referring patients to an alternative process that may or may not produce results is not my approach. I try to solve the problem at hand with what I know will work. Still, in all fairness, I encourage my patients to try other therapies if they have the inclination.

Ten-Minute Sleep Relief

Sleep deprivation should always be remedied by returning to adequate sleep patterns. On the other hand, if there is no way to completely make up for lost sleep, the next best natural remedy is to take a ten-minute afternoon nap each day. A number of famous people, including the late president John F. Kennedy, used catnaps successfully to boost endurance and energy. Studies published in the May 2001 issue of the journal *Sleep* show that longer naps tend to cause mental difficulties that are not encountered by the shorter naps. With ten-minute sleep relief, the limited sleep time prevents a deep sleep from which it is difficult to awaken. When you take a longer nap, you are likely to develop grogginess, headaches, depression, or other discomforts.

Deliberate Sleep Deprivation

Deliberate sleep deprivation is another way to treat insomnia. According to findings reported in a 2001 issue of the journal *Depression and Anxiety,* avoiding sleep for at least twenty-four hours is a recognized and formal way to reset the sleep cycle. Most of my patients refuse to do it, however, and those who have tried this approach have not experienced the type of recovery that is promised. I bring it to your attention mainly for informational value.

Drugs and Sleep

When I find it necessary to prescribe drugs to resolve sleep problems, I use the ones least likely to cause addiction. One is the over-the-counter sleep aid and antihistamine Benadryl, although I have found that its beneficial effect tends to wear off over time. The two prescription medications I use most are BuSpar (buspirone) and Atarax (hydroxyzine). BuSpar is non-addicting, safe, and effective in a fair number of patients. The second, Atarax, serves well as both a sleeping aid and an antihistamine. When allergies are part of the problem with either sleep or anxiety, Atarax is often helpful. This drug is frequently used as a children's medication. If these two don't work, I then resort to the prescription medication Restoril (temazepam), and suggest that patients take it once or twice a week while using nutrient sleeping aids on alternate nights.

For severe insomnia, I typically prescribe something like Restoril for a few days in the very beginning, knowing that my intention is for the patient to end up exclusively on nutrients. I have them take the medication so they'll have a standard for the level of sleep we must achieve through the nutritional approach. It also allows patients to enjoy the relief from anxiety that follows a deep restful sleep. Once they experience this, it's easier to motivate them to work toward that result.

Multiple Therapies

Recently, a patient complained that the prescribed sleeping medication was not extending her sleep for more than three hours a night. She said that the drug she was using was the best she and her doctor could come up with after a number of trials.

I left the woman on the medication, so as not to offend her doctor. But I added a nutrient, and her sleep time improved. When I added a second nutrient, her sleep improved more. Still, she was not getting an optimal night's sleep. Finally, I added a third nutrient to the formula and we hit the jackpot. It took three nutrients and one medication before she enjoyed a solid night's sleep.

In case you are worrying about the number of components necessary in this case, I must remind you that this woman's sleep deprivation was much more harmful than any drug and nutrient formula. Her fatigue disappeared, her memory returned, and, overall, she functioned much better while using the formula. We left the drug and nutrient combination in place because she was so satisfied. However, we could have continued experimenting until she was completely free of the medication, with the number of nutrients reduced.

One could argue that we should have tried meditation or some other self-help process instead of using all of these agents. This patient still has that option if she elects to pursue it. I used the tools I had at hand and stopped when she asked me to.

Pace Yourself

Because fatigue and lack of sleep are precipitating causes of acute anxiety and depression, you need to become aware of their impact. Here are some important rules I give to anxiety patients:

- Don't cut sleep because of a project. You must pace yourself on the project to avoid an attack of anxiety or depression.

- Don't allow yourself to become overly fatigued by taking on too much work. Pace your activities.
- Don't avoid food to the point of exhaustion. When you are tired, you may set off your emotional weaknesses if you go too long without eating.
- Don't forget that you have a weakness or weaknesses that will explode if not restrained by energy and the stabilizing influence of sleep.
- Train yourself to monitor your sleep and your energy levels. Head off any activity that will impinge on these two safety walls, which defend you against loss of emotional control.
- Aim yourself directly at the target of maturity. Forming more adaptive habits and traits is what I call *attaining maturity*. Some people call it developing integrity. What it really means is learning to trust your good judgment and good behavior. Good judgment leads to self-respect.

DR. HUNT'S HOLISTIC RX: GET CALMING SLEEP

Before I review the best natural remedies to resolve sleep problems, I want you to assess your sleep. This is important, as once you have an idea of the severity of the problem you'll be able to respond to appropriate treatment more rapidly.

I devised the Hunt's Sleep Scale below to help you rate your sleep. Using this scale, you can select the best description of how you sleep today—and for the next few weeks to see if your sleep is improving or worsening as you start the natural therapies. If your sleep worsens (higher number), you may need to change to a different natural dietary supplement. Or you may need to see your doctor for a prescribed medication. If the sleep improves (lower number), that's a good sign that the holistic program is working for you.

Hunt's Sleep Scale

Copy this sleep scale onto a piece of paper and make multiple copies. To find your sleep quotient on the scale, circle the number that reflects how you slept last night. On the copies you've made, circle a number each morning for three or four weeks until you find the right combination of nutrients to aid in good sleep.

1 = superb sleep 5 = average sleep
10 = worst sleep imaginable

1   2   3   4   5   6   7   8   9   10

Normally I ask patients to try each new remedy for at least a week before moving on to the next one. A week is sufficient for a reasonable trial. Once you've assessed your sleep consider the natural modalities that follow to improve it.

1 to 7 on the Scale: If you rated your sleep as 1 to 7 on the scale, you might consider a product called Body Enhancer. This over-the-counter medication contains the natural hormone melatonin and amino acids and is available at natural food stores or at www.anxietyanddepressionrelief.com (see Resources). The label recommendation is one tablespoon at bedtime. More than 50 percent of my patients who rate themselves between 1 and 7 on Hunt's Sleep Scale will achieve a good night's sleep using this product. In fact, I get this result even when I go no further in the questioning.

If the remedy just mentioned doesn't work or only works for part of the night, I ask more questions. If you awaken three to six times a night but drop back to sleep after a short while, I recommend adding 500 mg of tryptophan, which your doctor must prescribe. Alternatively, you might use 25 mg of 5-HTP as a substitute.

If you have a pattern of abruptly awakening once or twice during the night and can't return to sleep, I recommend keeping calcium and magnesium tablets by your bed and taking one or two when you awaken, at least 200 mg of each.

If you still need assistance in maintaining solid sleep, consider adding the natural hormone melatonin, discussed on pages 220–222, 3 to 12 mg at bedtime.

Trial and error is the only practical way of reaching success because there are no lab tests that will match patients to a particular remedy. Still, about 85 percent of the time I am able to avoid the use of drugs in a cooperative patient. Another 10 to 12 percent of the time, patients do well with mostly nutrients and the occasional use of medications. Four or 5 percent of the time, I must prescribe medications, and I can usually predict when this will be the case.

8 to 10 on the Scale: If you ranked your sleep difficulties from 8 to 10 on the scale, you might need some type of medication. Especially if you have a family history, your grandmother and mother both had insomnia, for instance, you might have a more serious metabolic sleep dysfunction that runs in families.

A number below 8 on the 10-point scale usually responds to an uncomplicated natural approach. A number over 8 might require a mixed approach using medications with nutrients. If drugs are necessary, trust your doctor to make the right decision for your case.

When your overall body chemistry has returned to a more normal state, you can consider reducing the nutrients (or medications). Still, these nutrients are important for long-term wellness and their usage is a positive health effect—not negative.

Keep in mind that other anxiety conditions can occur the same time you are tackling the sleep problem. As the other remedies in the book improve anxiety symptoms, your sleep problem will typically decline from 50 percent all the way down to zero.

Because everyone is so different, you may have to use trial and error to find the right combination of nutrients and medications, if needed, until you sleep like a baby. Sweet dreams!

DR. HUNT'S HOLISTIC RX FOR SLEEP PROBLEMS

It is important to remember that the following information represents examples of what I prescribe for my anxiety patients. I am not directly prescribing them for you, the reader. Examples of treatment are not a substitute for professional care where individualization is possible and necessary. Check with your doctor and ask if the following natural therapies might be used to increase calming sleep.

Insomnia or disturbed sleep
- 500 to 1,000 mg of the amino acid tryptophan at bedtime
- 25 mg of 5-hydroxytryptophan (5-HTP)
- 200 mg of calcium and magnesium each
- 3 to 12 mg of melatonin at bedtime

- Substitute: 1 tablespoon Body Enhancer at bedtime (see Resources)

Nocturnal pain
- 100 to 500 mg of methylsulfonomethane (MSM) before bedtime
- 250 to 500 mg of glucosamine sulfate

Panicky nights
- 100 to 500 mg of thiamine at bedtime
- Avoid alcohol, sugary snacks, and certain drugs such as decongestants or medications that contain caffeine
- 50 mg of potassium bicarbonate along with 1 scoop (provided in the jar) of glutathione powder
- Substitute: 2 baby aspirin, 1,000 mg of the amino acid acetyl carnitine, and 400 mg magnesium; add 25 mg of 5-HTP if needed

Night twitches
- 4 mg or more of the mineral manganese prior to bedtime
- 800 IU of vitamin E if needed
- 250 to 500 mg of the amino acid acetyl carnitine taken at bedtime if needed

Nocturnal acidity
- Eat a lightly salted piece of turkey or chicken before bedtime
- Keep bedroom cool
- Avoid sweets
- Buffered pH capsules from VAXA (see Resources)

Hypoglycemia
- Eat a lightly salted slice of chicken or turkey before going to bed
- Avoid sweets

Snoring or sleep apnea
- 100 to 200 mg of progesterone (prescription medication recommended for men only)

❦

Chapter 9

Step 5: Exercise to De-Stress

"My life is a never-ending treadmill," Lorna said. "With three teenagers, teaching full-time, and caring for my elderly mother, I feel like if I stop, I may never get up again. Sometimes, I lie in bed for hours at night thinking about everything I need to do yet there is never enough time or energy to get it all done—much less have time for myself."

Just hearing about Lorna's busy life made me feel anxious! I explained that her fast-paced life was causing unnecessary stress as she tried to be all things to all people. The anxiety she was feeling, along with an inability to sleep well at night, were warning signs that she wasn't responding to life's stressors in a healthy way.

The good news for Lorna was that she could successfully manage her stressful life by altering her response. In other words, instead of feeling escalating anxiety as all the many demands of life pile up, she needed to find a viable way to reduce this pent-up tension before her physical and emotional health was negatively affected. I shared with Lorna the exercise prescription in this chapter, and her life quickly took a turn for the better.

Ask anyone if they think that exercise improves mood and the majority of answers will be yes. A number of studies have confirmed this commonsense belief. For example, a study published in the August 2002 issue of *Scandinavian Journal of Medicine and Science in Sports* revealed that women who exercised, even as little as twice a week, had a more positive state of mental health. These scientists found that the difference between the emotional state of physically active women and inactive women, especially if there was depression, was significant. In a similar study, scientists at Brigham Young University concurred that working adults who participated in a moderate amount of physical activities were about half as stressed as nonparticipants. Another study on the effect of exercise on patients with major depression was presented in the April 2001 issue of the *British Journal of Sports Medicine*. In this study, researchers concluded that aerobic exercise produces substantial improvement in mood in patients with major depressive disorders in just a short time.

Exercise also appears to ease depression in those who worry excessively. In findings presented in June 2002 at the American Psychological Society's annual meeting in New Orleans, researchers concluded that chronic worriers appeared to be less likely to suffer depressive symptoms if they exercised than if they didn't exercise. While the study was performed on students during final exam week, researchers affirmed that the findings should apply to all worriers—and exercise is the treatment.

Exercise boosts the body's production of the brain's morphine-like pain relievers, called endorphins and enkephalins, which are associated with a happy, positive feeling. Endorphins also help to reduce anxiety, stress, and depression by restoring the body's neurochemical balance, which affects our emotional state. Not only does physical activity increase alpha waves in the brain, which are associated with relaxation and meditation, exercise also acts as a displacement defense mechanism for those who are stressed out.

If you have ever participated in a lengthy period of aerobic exercise or walked for several miles, perhaps you know the benefit of this displacement defense mechanism. It's not easy to worry about daily stresses when you are working your muscles physically. Your mind is focused on the activity—not the numerous problems you face each day. When you are more in control of your life after exercise, then excessive anxiety is less likely to transpire.

EXERCISE AND ANXIETY

If you are like many of my patients with an anxiety disorder, you are exhausted from sleepless nights and probably cringe when the word "exercise" is mentioned. After all, exercise demands energy—something you just don't have right now. Or maybe you identify with my patient Britt, a young woman who suffered with frequent panic attacks after being injured during a gymnastics stunt. Even though Britt was a passionate gymnast in high school and college, she developed a real phobia to any exercise after the accident for fear she might get hurt again. Britt reasoned that since the fall from the bars caused her injury and subsequent panic attacks, if she didn't move around much, she could avoid falling and the added anxiety. Wrong!

When patients like Lorna and Britt come to my clinic, one of the first recommendations I make is exercise. I explain that in almost every situation anxiety can be reduced—and even stopped completely—with regular movement and activity. Swimming, aerobics, playing tennis, walking, biking, and more can all help release the pent-up stress hormones in the body, helping you to feel more relaxed and less likely to become nervous or panicky.

Relieving the Pressure of Daily Stress

Have you ever accidentally dropped a carbonated drink can? When you pull the metal tab to open the shaken drink, it explodes. Now, try this. Carefully open the tab so just the smallest amount of carbonated fizz is released. When you open the pressurized can gradually over a longer period, the force is reduced and there is no explosion.

Try to imagine your body being similar to that can of soda. Your daily stress is the fizz or carbonation that activates when the can of soda is dropped. In this regard, it takes just a tiny amount of stress before your body reacts with the pumping fight-or-flight response (see page 57). When your stress is chronic, day after day, and you have not released the built-up adrenaline (a combination of epinephrine and norepinephrine), which makes your heart pump and muscles tense, then just like the shaken soda, you will explode. The explosion results in symptoms of high anxiety, panic attacks, fears, phobias, and worries, or hypertension, ulcers, or other chronic illness.

It does not have to be this way as there is a simple solution for this buildup of adrenaline. You have to let some fizz escape each day before it has a chance to burst and cause a cadre of emotional and physical problems. Exercise or moving around more each day will allow stress hormones to escape so they do not build up and wreak havoc with your mind and body.

The Science of Stress and Exercise

There are a number of reasons why exercise will help reduce anxiety, including the following:

• Exercise is the only known way to increase the number of mitochondria in the body's cells, and the cells' mitochondria make our energy. The more mitochondria you have, the more energy available for your needs, and more energy increases positive feelings.

• Exercise is an excellent way of releasing stored-up muscle tension. As tension is released, the muscles relax and so does the need to be on guard. All systems in the body will decompress.

• Exercise increases circulation and metabolism, which results in elevated energy and a sense of well-being. This consciousness of self-improvement reassures us of the correctness of our commitment.

• Exercise increases lymph flow and gastrointestinal passage, important for detoxification of waste materials, and results in improved energy and mood.

• Besides building the size and strength of muscles, exercise temporarily stores energy (not tension) in them. Stored muscular energy continually signals the brain that it is available for use (unlike the stored energy in fat cells). Young children are continually active because their youthful state taps into the constant feeling of available energy. Feeling this boundless supply of power, kids are constantly playful. For adults the new sense of power that comes with exercise reduces anxiety and fear.

De-Tensing Muscles

While anxiety starts in the mind, your muscles store it. Of course, popular medications can dim the production of anxiety, but pharmaceuticals have no influence on the muscles, what I call the "anxiety storage depot." It's logical then that if you could find a way to de-tense the muscles, to rid them of the bound-up energy, then your feelings of anxiety would be greatly reduced. Not surprisingly, this tensing and releasing of muscles is a well-known approach of traditional medicine. Simply review the many physical techniques that psychologists and physicians have developed to reduce anxiety and you will see a common thread: All such techniques work through one mechanism—muscle relaxation. Consider the following stress reduction therapies:

- progressive muscle relaxation
- hypnosis
- meditation
- massage
- biofeedback
- applying warm compresses to muscles

We doctors know that when the muscles relax so does anxiety. I tell my patients that a warm bath is like chicken soup for muscle tension!

USE DYNAMIC TENSION

One surefire and scientific way to reduce anxiety is to use dynamic tension, a method of discharging tension from muscle bundles and thereby dissipating anxiety. Dynamic tension costs nothing and yet it works nearly every time. There is one critical point to this exercise; it must be done correctly to be effective. Do the dynamic tension exercises several times a week to get used to how they are done. Then use them anytime you feel stressed or anxious.

A Warning About Dynamic Tension

Do not use this technique if you are epileptic, have had a stroke, or have hypertension, an irregular heart rhythm, or any other cardiovascular weakness. If in doubt, talk to your doctor.

Sean's Life Crisis and Anxiety

Sean was a perfectionist who allowed his anxiety problems to control his life. When this thirty-two-year-old software engineer lost his job a few weeks before his twins were born, Sean's perfect life turned to utter chaos. He coped with this stress by obsessing over his finances— from the bills he had to pay to his wife being unable to work for several months—and there were no easy answers. Sean said he stayed awake most nights worrying incessantly. Then the next day he could not function. Yet he knew he had to pull his life together and get a job to support his family.

I recommended that Sean learn the dynamic tension Push or Pull technique to get out his anxieties before he felt overwhelmed. I also suggested that he try 5-HTP, some B vitamins, and peppermint spray, if he felt panicked. Sean immediately vowed to do all of this and within a few weeks was back in control of his life and well-being. Once his unemployment crisis ended and he found another job, Sean felt more in control and was less anxious. He was grateful to know there were natural ways to stop and reverse anxiety before it engulfed him.

The Push or Pull Technique

The Push or Pull technique is a fast and effective way to overcome a fearful situation when you are caught unexpectedly with anxiety. This technique can be done quietly and surreptitiously and does not require special workout equipment. Your own body parts are used as "equipment."

With the Push or Pull, you put a pair of limbs such as your hands against each other. Alternatively, you can use some nearby object to push against or pull, such as a wall or pole if the object is anchored and stationary. If you're in a meeting or attending a function where you'd rather not draw attention to yourself, you can even use the armrest on a chair as your tool of deliverance. Another alternative is to use the seat of the chair you are sitting in, a wall you are near, a post nearby, the bottom or top of a desk.

With this dynamic tension exercise, it's important to remember that the more strength and power you put into this exercise, the quicker you will dissipate your anxiety.

Arm wrestle yourself. To get started with the Push or Pull technique, place your hands together, palm against palm with fingers interlocked, about eight inches in front of your mid-chest area in preparation for pitting the strength of one arm against the other. Keep your fists together firmly grasping each other and muster all the strength you can. Now shove one fist against the other with every ounce of strength you have in you. Each fist must be determined to defeat the other with a do-or-die attitude. While tensing the arms and hands in this struggle, you can include other muscles at the same time such as those in your shoulders, chest, neck, jaw, or abdomen.

Do a full round. I tell my patients to call each dynamic tension-relieving attempt a round, like in boxing or wrestling. Always take a deep breath before you start each Push or Pull round. Then, shove your hands and arms against themselves as hard as possible and for as long as possible. Watch the clock and make the first rounds last at least thirty seconds for best results. Try to extend that to more than a minute or even longer on subsequent rounds. Do a minimum of three or four rounds. Remember: The goal is to attain complete muscle exhaustion, and that usually takes more than three attempts.

When doing the Push or Pull, give it your all—and then some! Struggle as if your life depended on it, and stop only when you feel you have achieved complete muscle failure—not a second before. If you do the technique correctly, you will feel free of anxiety and completely relaxed. (Practically speaking, you will never reach every muscle fiber but you can reach most of the skeletal muscles where the largest cache of tension is stored.)

At the end of each Push or Pull round, feel the tension drain out of your body and fully experience the calmness. Usually by the third or fourth round, you will begin to feel warm and relaxed all over. After a series of rounds you should feel loose and relaxed, ready for a meeting, a presentation, or whatever the day will throw at you.

Here's another example to help you use the Push or Pull technique effectively. Say you are waiting for a job interview and you are wound-up, nervous, and worried that your nervousness will undermine a good presentation. I tell patients to go to a nearby restroom or empty room, face a wall, and brace their body with their hands while leaning on the wall. Now, take a deep breath and then shove your arms into the wall with enough strength to try to topple it altogether. After thirty seconds, stop, relax, and then do another round. The harder and longer you push, the more your bound-up anxiety is forced out of every muscle. Do a third round, and push even harder and longer. If you are doing this correctly, your nervousness will fade quickly, and you will breathe easier and feel more relaxed. Continue your rounds until you feel ready to tackle the interview (or other stressful situation).

Alternatively, you can pull against some object like a post or a pillar. Clasp both hands around the post, brace your feet at the foot of the post, take a deep breath and don't stop pulling until you feel your muscles giving way. You can push or pull against any solidly set object—but the energy necessary for success must be your top effort.

Bob's Midnight Struggle

Forty-six-year-old Bob explained to me how he had benefited from the Push or Pull technique. Bob was facing some difficult personal problems, more than enough to keep him from sleeping. Even when he was able to fall asleep, it usually did not last for more than two hours before he was awakened in a near-panic state. While on a business trip, Bob could not obtain any of my recommended natural sleeping remedies, so he tried the Push or Pull technique.

Lying in bed, Bob put his palms together in front of him and locked his fingers. He then shoved his hands against each other with terrific force, trying to include the muscles of his neck, face, shoulders, abdomen, and legs. He was determined to continue pushing, one hand against the other, until there was not a drop of strength left in him.

Bob's first round of Push or Pull lasted just over two minutes. Bob worked so hard at the Push or Pull that he fell back sweating and panting. Nevertheless, he didn't give up! He decided his first effort was below his real capabilities, so he locked his hands together again for another round. Bob swore to himself that this time he would not stop until every muscle was completely exhausted. While he surpassed his first effort, he still did not feel it was his best.

Bob then checked himself for anxiety and worry. He felt somewhat relaxed, but there was still some residual anxiety. Once more, he applied every drop of his remaining energy to the process and ended the session completely exhausted and unable to continue. A minute or two later, Bob fell asleep and awoke refreshed seven hours later.

The next three days were the most carefree and tranquil days of Bob's adult life. Nothing bothered him. The problems he faced had not disappeared, but they were not haunting him or influencing his mood and outlook on life. Bob continued the Push or Pull technique daily and did extra rounds when he felt anxious. Like all things in life, his current problems eventually disappeared into the past.

Bob realized what I've told all my patients—if you give full commitment to learning and using the Push or Pull technique, it will amaze you with anxiety-relieving results.

GET REGULAR EXERCISE TO DE-STRESS

When I first met Claudia, she had suffered with high anxiety, fears, and worries for most of her adult life. This forty-three-year-old fashion designer had resorted to working at home because she could no longer endure the stress of driving to an office and meeting with clients. When Claudia drove to the grocery store, she had to pull over on the side of the road several times to calm herself down. If anyone came to her door unexpectedly, she would hide in her bedroom and pretend she was not home for fear it was someone who might harm her.

As we talked about her medical history, Claudia admitted that she had tried everything to resolve her anxiety—from tranquilizers to antidepressants to herbal therapies, homeopathy, and even hypnosis. Nothing seemed to help. After a while, she quit taking any of the prescribed drugs because they made her so exhausted that she could not work.

When I asked how often she exercised, Claudia said, "Not at all." She explained her fear of having anxiety during exercise and was very guarded in where she went, so going to a fitness center was out of the question.

Even though Claudia had such negative feelings about exercise, I explained that the anxious tension she felt was in every fiber of every muscle in her body. Therefore, every fiber of every muscle that she had access to had to be drained before she could be completely free of anxiety. Increased exercise and activity was an easy way to feel relief of this bottled-up tension and anxiety that haunted her. Exercise might even allow her to reclaim her active life again. I convinced Claudia to start the exercise Rx in this step and, within a few weeks, she was amazed by how much she had greatly reduced her anxiety and fears.

On a side note, after six months using my 5-step holistic

program, Claudia came to the clinic for a follow-up evaluation. She said she was taking no medication, sleeping through the night, and was dating someone in her condominium association. She even joined the Y and started a low-impact aerobics class with other women.

There is no question about the value of exercise for weight loss or prevention of heart disease. We know that exercise helps to build strong bones and prevent osteoporosis. Nevertheless, most people are unaware that exercise is vital to reduce anxiety disorders. Years of comprehensive studies indicate that aerobic exercise training has antidepressant effects and helps to protect against detrimental consequences of stress. It does not take much exercise to modulate mood. In a large Finnish study of 3,403 participants (1,856 women and 1,547 men), age twenty-five to sixty-four, published in the January 2000 issue of *Preventive Medicine,* researchers found that those individuals who exercised at least two or three times a week experienced significantly less depression, anger, cynical distrust, and stress than those who exercised less frequently or not at all.

While most of my patients benefit from a regular exercise program, there are a few who claim that exercise worsens their anxiety symptoms. These compulsive exercisers keep working out harder and longer, thinking that more will give them better results. In doing so, working out too much can sometimes cause fatigue, sluggishness, and increased anxiety. Those with social phobia may refrain from group exercise for fear of being exposed to unfamiliar surroundings such as the local Y or fitness center. In that case, I encourage them to exercise at home using a treadmill or stationary bike.

However, moderate exercise has tremendous overall health benefits. It makes sense that if you experience optimal health, you feel better, have a more positive outlook on life, and your anxiety will lessen.

Always Warm Up

Always warm your muscles before you exercise. Walk or march in place or climb up and down a flight of stairs slowly for a few minutes before you engage in any exercise activity. Focus on regular breathing during your warm-up. This warm-up causes an increased circulation of blood to the muscles and helps reduce stiffness and prevents injury.

Aerobics Keep Muscles Healthy

I recommend to my patients that they add aerobic or conditioning exercises to their daily to-do list. This includes any exercise that increases heart rate and keeps it higher for a certain period. Aerobic and conditioning exercises help your heart and muscles use oxygen more efficiently, and muscles that frequently receive oxygen-rich blood stay healthier. Make sure you warm up before any exercise and then slowly and gradually increase the movements.

Conditioning exercise does not have to take your breath away to be effective! Just get up off the couch and move around more—walk, climb stairs, swim, ride a bike, dance, walk your dog, or play with your kids or grandkids. Conditioning exercise does not have to be vigorous or continuous. In findings published in the July 2001 issue of *Health Psychology*, researchers found that after just ten minutes of conditioning exercise, study participants had improvements in vigor, energy, and total mood. Try just ten minutes of movement three times daily to reduce anxiety and increase well-being.

LeeAnne's Panic Attacks

LeeAnne, a twenty-nine-year-old attorney, felt her career was over when she started having panic attacks for no reason. Whether in the midst of doing legal research in a quiet library or making a presentation to a jury, she'd start shaking, sweating, and having heart palpitations. In fact, the symptoms were so violent, she often felt as if she were having a heart attack.

I suggested that LeeAnne start exercising daily to help reduce the stress hormones in the body, which can trigger sudden panic attacks. She also stopped drinking caffeinated beverages and began taking magnesium, 5-HTP, the amino acid L-theanine, and melatonin at bedtime to assist with sleep. LeeAnne used the peppermint spray Body Control several times a day when she felt panicked. Within a few weeks, she felt more relaxed than she had in years and her panic attacks decreased. After using this natural regimen for three months, LeeAnne reported having no more panic attacks at all.

Yoga Eases Body Tension

Yoga is a popular way to condition the body. This ancient form of exercise is also an excellent way to relieve anxiety and muscle tension. Yoga helps you to slow down and focus on the moment instead of stressing about all the things on your to-do list. The various yoga postures, if done correctly, can aid in calming the mind, which in turn relaxes the muscles in the body.

Many studies have been done on the benefits of yoga to the mind and body. For instance, in an effort to observe the beneficial effect of yogic practices on young trainees, findings published in the January 2001 issue of the *Indian Journal of Physiology and Pharmacology* showed improvement in various psychological parameters like reduction in anxiety and depression and a better mental function after yogic practices.

Practicing yoga when you are feeling tense or anxious may help reduce stress no matter what the source. With any type of yoga, you may find great benefit from the physical postures (asanas) to alleviate aching muscles, concentration exercises (dharana) to overcome dwelling on your personal problems, and meditation (dhyana) to help you focus on the present instead of ruminating about daily worries.

Yoga can help clear your head and allow you to focus on the here and now instead of what might be—or what might have been. Instead of giving into negative thoughts, you will learn to "feel the breath" and calm the mind with yoga poses and this will lead to feelings of inner peace. Many yogis believe we hold emotions deep in the body with the outward signs of hunched shoulders, tight lips, and furrowed brows. Through yoga, you can tap into these patterns of chronic tightness, release the muscles, and begin to heal the emotional wounds.

DR. HUNT'S HOLISTIC RX: EXERCISE TO DE-STRESS

If you are already exercising, good for you! The only question is whether it is enough or too much. Too little exercise maintains a growing weakness. On the other hand, too much exercise will actually start to break down muscular tissues. Time must be allowed between sessions to repair wear and tear as well as to deal with free radical buildup that occurs during exercise, especially prolonged or intense exercise.

Thirty minutes of exercise three times a week is the absolute minimum. If you prefer to exercise in the privacy of your home, consider purchasing an electronic treadmill, StairMaster, or stationary bicycle. Set the equipment in front of your television and watch an old movie or funny video while you work out. Walk the dog before and after work, take the stairs instead of elevators, and park at the end of the lot when you go shopping to increase your daily physical exercise time. Swimming is the best all-in-one exercise, as it conditions the muscles, exercises the lungs (and expands them, important to the lower lung area, which gets the least expansion), thus improving blood oxygenation. It heightens, stretches, and strengthens tendons and helps to boost cardiovascular endurance.

Along with increasing your stretching, conditioning, and strengthening exercises each day, I want you to learn and perfect the dynamic tension Push or Pull technique and become acquainted with its benefits.

Once you start this exercise step, you will notice a decrease in anxiety symptoms. But if you stop exercising, you will lose the benefits you were building. This step is not a short-term Band-Aid but a long-term commitment to achieving optimal emotional and physical health.

Sample 2-Week Exercise Rx

Monday: 30-minute walk with friends
Tuesday: 10 minutes of resistance machines at the Y; yoga class
Wednesday: 20-minute swim followed by stretches

Thursday: 10 minutes of resistance machines at the Y; water aerobics class

Friday: Household and gardening chores

Saturday: 20-minute swim followed by stretches

Sunday: 30-minute bike ride

Monday: 30-minute walk on indoor treadmill (done in 2 sessions of 15 minutes each)

Tuesday: 10 minutes of strengthening exercises using free weights; 1 hour gardening

Wednesday: 30-minute bike ride

Thursday: 10 minutes of resistance machines at the Y; stretching class

Friday: 30-minute walk during lunch hour

Saturday: 10 minutes of resistance machines at the Y; yoga class

Sunday: 3 hours gardening

Chapter 10

A Final Word: You *Can* Control Your Anxiety

You may be thinking, "After living with anxiety, phobias, and panic attacks for so many years, there is no natural therapy that can help me feel more in control." I'm out to prove you wrong, and, at the same time, help you stop or reverse your problems with anxiety.

I hope you have gained additional insight into the different types of anxiety disorders. Understanding the signs and symptoms of common problems such as generalized anxiety disorder, phobias, panic attacks, obsessive-compulsive disorder, acute stress reaction, and post-traumatic stress disorder can help you narrow down your specific problem and help your doctor in making the diagnosis.

As you have read in this book, there is no one set treatment for anxiety. Because each person's experience with anxiety is unique, the treatment will vary as well. Some patients need medications to feel calm; others find that my multidisciplinary approach helps to resolve anxiety; still others will use a combination approach of medications and natural therapies. Talk to your doctor about the therapies that are best for you.

My 5-step holistic program is not meant to be a stopgap or temporary solution for your specific anxiety problem. Rather, this program should be fully discussed with your doctor to see if it can become a part of your daily life for years to come. Following the program is a lifestyle process, not an end in itself. Changing behaviors over time that you may have followed for decades takes continual commitment on your behalf.

Again, I remind you that getting an accurate diagnosis is a critical piece of the anxiety puzzle. It's important to talk with a health care professional about your signs and symptoms, medical history, and family history to see what type of problem you have. When your doctor has all the facts, he or she can order laboratory tests, if needed, and then pinpoint the problem, make the diagnosis, and prescribe effective treatment, whether pharmaceuticals, nutrients, lifestyle changes, or a combination of these modalities.

Because you are not my patient, I cannot prescribe any therapies for your situation. But I can share with you what has worked for thousands of the men and women who come to my clinic. A few of these patients still take medications. Some use medications in conjunction with the natural therapies and lifestyle changes. But the majority of my patients rely strictly on the nutrients and lifestyle habits to help them reduce and even end anxiety and reclaim a relaxed and normal life.

Again, review the material in this book. Then if your doctor agrees, you can join the thousands of men and women who have learned to manage their anxiety disorders naturally and are enjoying full, unlimited lives again.

Glossary

─────── ⚭ ───────

ACTH-cortisol pathway—ACTH is the hormone released from the pitutary gland in the brain to stimulate release of hormones from the outer layer (the cortex) of the adrenal gland. Cortisol is a natural steroid that is secreted by this area under stress to combat stress; however, it can be toxic if secreted too long or too profusely.

Adrenergic system—Includes adrenaline from the adrenal gland and neurotransmitters related to the sympathetic nervous system (SNS) and the nerves related to the sympathetic nervous system itself.

Amygdala—An important nucleus of cells found at the base of the temporal lobe (in the basal ganglia) of the brain that is essential for emotional control and emotional memories. It is sometimes called the fear center of the brain.

Anterior cingulate cortex—A long curved group of nerve fibers that, among other things, connects the thalamus and hippocampus to the frontal area of the brain. The front part of this well-marked group of fibers near the cortex of the brain is called the anterior part.

Anterior insula—An oval region deep within a fissure on the frontal part of the cerebral cortex. The area is active during anxiety.

Arrhythmia—An irregular heartbeat.

Autonomic nervous system—A system of nerves that operates autonomously, normally outside the control of the conscious. It is divided into the sympathetic and parasympathetic systems.

Axon—A single arm or extension of a nerve that conducts nerve impulses away from the cell.

Basal ganglia—The gray matter of the brain just under the thalamus. An area very much associated with anxiety.

Biorhythm—An innate periodicity of an organism's physiological process, such as the sleep-wake cycle.

Blood brain barrier—A membrane surrounding the brain, made up of glial cells, that acts as a filter against allowing entrance of large undesirable molecules and most ions.

Brain stem—The topmost area of the spinal cord, which expands out like the knob at the top of a walking stick. The brain sits directly on top of it.

Dr. Johanna Budwig—A German physician who did considerable clinical and laboratory research on lipids and fatty acids for nutritional-medical applications. She wrote a number of books citing her findings, all of which are in German. Her results are often referred to by American writers.

Calcium channel—A passageway through a cell wall that relates specifically to ionic calcium.

Central nervous system—The brain plus the spinal cord.

Cingulate gyrus, cingulate area, cingulate cortex—A long curved group of nerve fibers that, among other things, connects the thalamus and hippocampus to the frontal area of the brain. *Cortex* refers to the part near the front (anterior), *gyrus* and *area* refer to the body or main curving group of fibers. This group of nerves connects the feeling, orienting part of the brain to the thinking area in the front of the brain.

Circadian rhythms or cycles—An internal biological clock that produces cycles or rhythms related to a twenty-four-hour time frame.

Cortical processing areas—Various areas of the brain that are responsible for processing conscious information.

Corticotropin releasing factor—A hormone released from a higher level in the brain instructing the pituitary gland to release ACTH, a hormone that will then stimulate hormone release from the cortex of the adrenal gland. This is much more active during stress.

Dendrites—Branching, treelike extensions from a nerve that transport nerve impulses toward the nerve body. They accept chemical messages from other nerves.

Downregulated—A receptor on a nerve that has become indifferent or insensitive to the amount of compatible neurotransmitters in its vicinity.

Dysmorphic ideation—A persistent belief that the individual's body is seriously flawed in one or more ways. This may quickly rise to the level of a delusion.

Eosinophil—A type of white blood cell (part of our immune system) or leukocyte that very often increases in number during allergic symptoms.

Flavonoid—A natural substance derived from plants that has a large variety of beneficial health effects. As is related to this book, its most positive effect is on allergy.

Frontal lobe—The front part of the brain. It is often called the executive part because it is the area where most intellectual decisions and planning take place.

Hippocampus—A curved ridge on the lateral ventricles in the center of the brain that is part of the limbic or emotional center. This structure plays a critical role in memory storage and retrieval.

Homeostasis—An innate system in humans and other animals responsible for maintaining normal physiological balance of the internal environment.

Hypothalamus—A structure in the center of the brain that controls heart rate, hunger, sex drive, thirst, aggressiveness, pleasure, temperature, and a generalized response to stress of all kinds.

Ion channel gatekeepers—Ion channels look like tiny floating protein donuts on a sea of oil. The hole or pore in the "donut" is actually the beginning of a passage through the cell wall, which is chiefly made of oil. Molecular guards, made of protein, patrol the gate, allowing only the ions they recognize through the tunnel to the inside of the cell.

Limbic system—An area, deep in the brain, that is important to all the intense emotions we feel. The limbic lobe or limbic system comes from the Latin word *limbus*, which describes a circle or ring of neurons that forms a border or cap around the topmost part of the brain stem. This system is just as important to survival as the expression of like and dislike through emotions.

Lipooxygenase—An enzyme related to inflammation through its effects on the eicosanoid system. Eicosanoids are lipid mediators of inflammation that are derived from arachidonic acid, a polyunsaturated fatty acid. A well-balanced intake of essential fatty acids will keep this system under good control.

Locus ceruleus—A cluster of nerves lying near the brain's fourth ventricle but within the brain stem, which has been found to relate to fear and anxiety. Any increase in activity in this center will cause anxiety, while reductions of activity in this area will decrease anxiety.

Mast cell degranulation—Mast cells (a type of white blood cell) are widely distributed around the body and are usually found adjacent to small blood vessels. These cells are loaded with very active, inflammation-generating, basophilic granules. In addition to causing an inflammation, they release histamine, which passes through the circulation to cause an allergic reaction elsewhere as well as at the original location.

Master oscillator—To oscillate is to move to and fro to create a wave frequency that may be used to transmit information or to control anything that responds to that frequency. The master oscillator is the control center for all other oscillators.

Microtubule event—Microtubules are dynamic, ever-changing polymers that are critical to cellular functions. These tubules are one-cell-thick tubes that occur in vast numbers within mammalian cells. They function as transporters of molecules, communication networks, stabilizers for cell structure, and for dozens of other uses. Damage to this system is a severe blow to cellular health. A microtubule event is simply a tubule performing one of its important tasks.

Narcolepsy—A sleep disorder characterized by recurring episodes of unavoidable sleep during the day and disturbed sleep at night. It appears to be genetically determined.

Neuron—The principal information-carrying unit of the nervous system. The three parts of the neuron, or nerve cell, are the cell body, the dendrites (which accept information into the neuron), and the axon (which transmits information from the neuron).

Neuropeptide—A large molecule composed of multiple amino acids that specifically acts on nerve and nerve-related tissues.

Neurotransmitter—A chemical released by one neuron to communicate with an adjacent neuron. Examples include: gamma-aminobutyric acid (GABA), serotonin, dopamine, epinephrine (adrenaline), and norepinephrine.

Orbitofrontal cortex—Located in the front part of the brain, this center functions to integrate sight, smell, taste, and touch. Its association with the cingulate system creates an additional aspect of reward or punishment. This area of the brain evaluates what it senses, good or bad, and passes that information on to the emotional centers for their reaction.

Paralimbic—An area of the brain adjacent to the limbic system that has been found, through SPECT scan studies, to be active during emotional responses.

Parietal cortex—A location on the cortex of the brain that becomes activated by tasks related to visual motor control, attention, and eye movements.

Phospholipase A—A calcium-dependent enzyme that is related to inflammation.

Platelet aggregation—Means blood coagulation. Platelets (thrombocytes) are the primary blood-clotting system for the blood. This is good if you cut yourself but could cause a stroke or heart attack if the system becomes too sensitive.

Precursor—A molecule or chemical substance that is utilized in the construction of a larger molecule. A substance from which another is derived.

Psychotropic drug—A drug that is specifically designed to treat some form of mental illness.

Receptor—A protein structure on a cell wall (in this instance a nerve cell) that binds to a specific factor such as a drug, hormone, antigen, or neurotransmitter from which a reaction ensues within the cell.

Reticular activating system—A center, located in the midbrain, that alerts us and maintains our attention. It is a complex collection of neurons that integrates signals from our internal and external environment.

Reuptake—Recapturing a chemical factor such as a neurotransmitter that was originally held by the nerve cell.

SNS—Sympathetic nervous system.

Sulfhydryl group—See thiol.

Synapse—The membrane-to-membrane contact of one nerve cell to another in order to pass messages between the two. In most cases there is a fifteen- to fifty-nanometer gap between the membranes. Chemical neurotransmitters carry the messages across the gap.

Temporal lobe—Contains part of the limbic system, the amygdala, and the hippocampus, and therefore is closely associated with fear, emotions, and memory of events. Through the temporal lobe the sensations of sight and sound reach the amygdala (fear center).

Thalamus—An organ in the center of the brain sitting on top of the brain stem that transmits and integrates sensory impulses.

Thiol (SH) group—A molecule composed of sulfur, hydrogen, and frequently carbon. This chemical combination has been therapeutic for skin diseases as well as metabolic problems.

Trichotillomania—Constantly pulling of one's hair.

Ultradian—Referring to biological rhythms occurring more frequently than every twenty-four hours.

Upregulated—A receptor on a nerve that has become extremely oversensitive or over-reactive to the amount of compatible neurotransmitters in its vicinity.

Working memory—Sometimes called short-term memory. Stimuli that have been recognized and registered are temporarily stored in a holding process to be recycled over and over during a planning or problem-solving situation. These memories may or may not be turned into long-term memories.

Resources

WHERE TO FIND RECOMMENDED SUPPLEMENTS, ALTERNATIVE THERAPIES, AND TESTING LABS

Most common nutrients are available at your natural food store. If you cannot find the recommended supplements or therapies locally, check with the following places:

- Body Enhancer (an excellent sleep aid) www.anxiety anddepressionrelief.com
- Body Control (an oral anti-anxiety peppermint spray) www.anxietyanddepressionrelief.com
- Mind at Work (an energy booster) www.anxietyand depressionrelief.com
- Nutrients such as zinc, thiamine, powdered inositol, DHEA, valerian, passionflower, colostrum, or other natural dietary supplements—www.vitaminshoppe.com
- Seasilver: www.seasilver.com. This product contains vitamins, minerals, amino acids, and enzymes to support the immune system.
- Celtic Sea Salt

The Grain and Salt Society
9300 Skyway
Paradise, California 95969
916-872-5800
www.celtic-seasalt.com

- Body Relief (a magnesium/calcium anti-anxiety aid) www.anxietyanddepressionrelief.com
- Body Biobalance (balanced essential oils) customerservice@bodybio.com
- Candida stool testing
Great Smokies Diagnostic Laboratories
63 Zillicoa Street
Asheville, NC 28801
800-522-4762
www.gsdl.com
- Analysis of antioxidant status
SpectraCell Laboratories
7051 Portwest Drive, #100
Houston, TX 77024
800-227-5227
www.spectracell.com
- Blood biopsy fatty acid analysis
Patricia Kane, Ph.D.
Haverford Wellness Center
2010 Westchester Pike
Philadelphia, PA 19083
610-924-0600
fax: 610-924-0625
kbraccia@juno.com
- To find a local educational psychologist
American Psychological Association
750 First Street N.E.

Washington, DC 20002
800-374-2721
www.apa.org

- SPECT imaging departments are found in most hospitals, especially teaching hospitals. Here are some contacts:

The Amen Clinic Newport Beach
4019 Westerly Place, Suite 100
Newport Beach, CA 92660
949-266-3700

The Amen Clinic Fairfield
350 Chadbourne Road
Fairfield, CA 94585
707-429-7181
www.amenclinic.com

- Amino acid testing
Metametrix Clinical Laboratory
4855 Peachtree Industrial Boulevard
Norcross, GA 30092
800-221-4640
www.metametrix.com

- The gastro test—available through physicians, chiropractors, naturopaths, and other health care specialists. This is relatively inexpensive compared to intubation or other current tests. The procedure is painless and results are available fifteen minutes after the test is completed. Older individuals may be suffering marginal malnutrition as a result of lack of sufficient gastric acid and not know it, so this test will be excellent for them. If your present health care provider is not familiar with the test, ask them to contact:

HDC Corporation
  628 Gibralter Court
  Milpitas, CA 95035
  800-227-8162
  www.hdccorp.com
- Buffered pH capsules
  VAXA
  4010 State Street
  Tampa, FL. 33609
  www.vaxa.com
- For information on the StrengthsQuest Program, a thirty-minute personal assessment test, see www.strengthquest.com.
- Alternative care treatment for the more extreme forms of mental illness
  Safe Harbor
  P.O. Box 37
  Sunland, CA 91041
  818-890-1862
- For a superb nutritional genius
  Diana Noland, Registered Dietitian
  1834 West Burbank Boulevard
  Burbank, CA 91506
  818-840-8098
- For Dr. Hunt's bimonthly newsletter www.anxietyand depressionrelief.com.

PROFESSIONAL ORGANIZATIONS

American Academy of Environmental Medicine
  7701 East Kellogg, #625
  Wichita, KS 67207

316-684-5500
fax: 316-684-5709
www.aaem.com

American College for Advancement in Medicine
23121 Verdugo Drive, #204
Laguna Hills, CA 92653
800-532-3688
fax: 949-455-9679
www.acam.org

American College of Nutrition
300 South Duncan Avenue, #225
Clearwater, FL 33755
727-446-6086
fax: 727-446-6202
www.amcollnutr.org

American Holistic Medical Association
12101 Menaul Boulevard, NE, #C
Albuquerque, NM 87112
505-292-7788
fax: 505-293-7582
www.holisticmedicine.org

International College of Integrative Medicine
333 La Grange Road, Suite 7
La Grange Park, IL 60526
708-579-1772
fax: 708-579-9176
www.icimed.com

COMPOUNDING PHARMACIES

There are two types of pharmacies in the U.S.: standard pharmacies and compounding pharmacies. Regular pharmacies basically count pills from drug companies. Compounding pharmacies require special licenses to make medicines in any special way a doctor recommends (i.e., an antibiotic in a suppository). All natural hormones must be created as special orders for each individual and are not off-the-shelf items. Natural hormones require the use of a compounding pharmacy since regular drug stores are unable to fill the prescription. Compounding pharmacies generally know all of the local alternative care physicians and so become a resource for anyone searching for such a doctor.

The following companies have lists of doctors who use hormone balancing with natural hormones as well as practice alternative medicine. The doctors listed are from all parts of the nation.

ApothéCure
    13720 Midway Road, #109
    Dallas, TX 75244
    800-969-6601
    www.apothecure.com

College Pharmacy
    3505 Austin Bluffs Parkway, #101
    Colorado Springs, CO 80918
    800-888-9358
    www.collegepharmacy.com

Kronos
    3675 South Rainbow Boulevard, #103
    Las Vegas, NV 89103

800-723-7455
www.kronospharmacy.com

Lakeside Pharmacy
4632 Highway 58 North
Chattanooga, TN 37416
800-523-1486
lakeside@unipharm.com

Panorama Pharmacy
6744 Balboa Boulevard
Lake Balboa, CA 91406
800-247-9767
www.panoramapharmacy.com

Women's International Pharmacy
12012 North 111 Avenue
Youngtown, AZ 85363
800-279-5708
www.womensinternational.com

References

Acuna-Castroviejo D, Martin M, Macias M, Escames G, Leon J, Khaldy H, Reiter RJ. (2001, March). Melatonin, mitochondria, and cellular bioenergetics. *J Pineal Res,* 30(2):65–74.

Agren G, Thiblin I, Tirassa P, Lundeberg T, Stenfors C. (1999, May). Behavioural anxiolytic effects of low-dose anabolic androgenic steroid treatment in rats. *Physiol Behav,* (3):503–9.

Aikey JL, Nyby JG, Annuth DM, James PJ. (2002, December). Testosterone rapidly reduces anxiety in male house mice. *Horm Behav,* 42(4)448–60.

Airapetiants MG, Levshina IP, Shuikin NN. (2000, March/April). The correction of the manifestations of a neurosis-like state in white rats by using the vitamin complex Aekol. *Zh Vyssh Nev Deiat Im I P Pavlova,* 50(2):274–80.

Aldans SG, Sutton LD, Jacobson BH, Quirk MG. (1996, February). Relationships between leisure-time physical activity and perceived stress. *Percept Mot Skills,* 82(1):315–21.

Arnold PD, Richter MA. (2001, November). Is obsessive-compulsive disorder an autoimmune disease? *CMAJ,* 13;165(10): 1353–58.

Arushanian EB, Beier EV. (1998, March/April). The participation of the dorsal hippocampus in the anti-anxiety action of melatonin and diazepam. *Eksp Klin Farmakol,* 61(2):13–6.

Bahrke MS, Yesalis CE, Wright JE. (1992, November/December). Psychological and behavioral effects of endogenous testosterone and anabolic-androgenic steroids. *Am J Sports Med,* 20(6):717–24.

Baker ER, Best RG, Manfredi RL, Demers LM, Wolf GC. (1995, March). Efficacy of progesterone vaginal suppositories in alleviation of nervous symptoms in patients with premenstrual syndrome. *J Assist Reprod Genet,* 12(3):205–9.

Balzola FA, Boggio-Bertinet D. (1996, March). The metabolism of glutamine. *Minerva gastroenterol Dietol,* 42(1):17–26.

Benca RM. (2001). Consequences of insomnia and its therapies. *J Clin Psychiatry;* 62 Suppl 10:33–38.

Benjamin J, Levine J, Fux M, Levy D, Belmaker RH. (1995, July). Double-blind, placebo-controlled, crossover trial of inositol treatment for panic disorder. *Am J. Psychiatry,* 152(7):1084-86.

Benton D, Fordy J, Haller J. (1995, February). The impact of long-term vitamin supplementation on cognitive functioning. *Psychopharmacology,* 117(3):298–305.

Benton D, Griffiths R, Haller J. (1997, January). Thiamine supplementation mood and cognitive functioning. *Psychopharmacology,* 129(1):66–71.

Benton D, Haller J, Fordy J. (1995). Vitamin supplementation for 1 year improves mood. *Neuropsychobiology,* 32(2):98–105.

Bhattacharya SK, Mitra SK. (1991, August). Anxiolytic activity of Panax genseng roots: an experiential study. *J Ethnopharmacol,* 34(1):87–92.

Birchall H, Brandon S, Taub N. (2000, June). Panic in a general practice population: prevalence, psychiatric comorbidity and associated disability. *Soc Psychiatry Psychiatr Epidem,* 35(6):235–41.

Blaschoko S, Zilker T, Forstl H. (1999, April). Idiopathic environmental intolerance (IPI)—formerly multiple chemical sensitivity

(MCS)—from the psychiatric perspective. *Fortschr Neurol Psychiatr*, 67(4):175–87.

Bockova E, Hronek J, Kolomaznik M, Polackova J, Curdova NO. (1992, August). Potentiation of the effects of anxiolytics with magnesium salts. *Cesk Psychiatr*, 88(3–4):141–44.

Borges CR, Geddes T, Watson JT, Kuhu DM. (2003, January). Dopamine biosynthesis is regulated by Glutathionylation. Potential mechanism of tyrosine hydrxylast inhibition during oxidative stress. *J Biol Chem*, 31;278(5):295–302.

Bouyer M, Bagdassarian S, Chaabanne S, Mullet E. (2001, June). Personality correlates of risk perception. *Risk Anal*, 21(3):457–65.

Brady KT. (1997). Posttraumatic stress disorder and comorbidity: recognizing the many faces of PTSD. *J Clin Psychiatry*, 58 Suppl 9:12–15.

Braner RB, Stangl M, Siewert JR, Pfab R, Becker K. (2003, February). Acute liver failure after administration of the herbal tranquilizer Kava-Kava (*Piper methysticum*). *J Clin Psy*, 64:2.

Brunello N, Davidson JR, Deahl M, Kessler RC, Mendlewicz J, Racagni G, Shalev AY, Zohar J. (2001). Postraumatic stress disorder: diagnosis and epidemiology, cormorbidity and social consequences, biology and treatment. *Neuropsychobiology*, 43(3):150–62.

Cain CK, Blouin AM, Barad M. (2002, October). L-type voltage-gated calcium channels are required for extinction, but not for acquisition or expression, of conditional fear in mice. *J Neurosci*, 15;22(20):9113–21.

Cassano GB, Pini S, Saettoni M, Dell'Osso L. (1999, March). Multiple anxiety disorder comorbidity in patients with mood spectrum disorders with psychotic features. *Am J Psychiatry*, 156(3):474–76.

Cauffield JS, Forbes HJ. (1999, May/June). Dietary supplements used in the treatment of depression, anxiety and sleep disorders. *Lippincott's Prim Care Pract*, 3:290–304.

Cline MA, Ochoa J, Torebjork HE. (1989, June). Chronic hyperalgesia and skin warming caused by sensitized C nociceptors. *Brain*, 112(pt 3):621–47.

Coghlan HC, Natello G. (1991). Erythrocyte magnesium in symptomatic patients with primary mitral valve prolapse: relationship to symptoms, mitral leaflet thickness, joint hypermobility and autonomic regulation. *Magnes Trace Elem*, (2–4):205–14.

Costello EJ, Mustillo S, Erkanli A, Keeler G, Angold A. (2003, August). Prevalence and development of psychiatric disorders in childhood and adolescence. *Arch Gen Psychiatry*, 60(8):837–44.

Cutolo M, Seriolo B, Villaggio B, Pizzorni C, Craviotto C, Suli A. (2002, June). Androgens and estrogens modulate the immune and inflammatory responses in rheumatoid arthritis. *Ann NY Acad Sci*, 966:131–42.

Danion JM, et al. (1989). Impairment in long term Benzodiazepine users. *Pharmacology*, 99:238–243.

Davidson JR, Connor KM, Sutherland SM. (1998). Panic disorder and social phobia: current treatments and new strategies. *Clev Clin J Med*, 65 Suppl 1:8139–44.

Davis S. (2001, March). Testosterone deficiency in women. *J Reprod. Med*, 46(3 Suppl):291–96.

Day R, Gido P, Helmus T, Fortier J, Roth T, Koshorek G, Rosenthal L. (2001, March). Self-reported levels of sleepiness among subjects with insomnia. *Sleep Med.* (2):153–57.

DeJongh A, Van Den Oord HJ, Ten Broeke E. (2002, December). Efficacy of eye movement desensitization and reprocessing in the treatment of specific phobias: Four single-case studies on dental phobia. *J Clin Psychol*, 58(12):1489–503.

De Sonza MC, Walker AF, Robinson PA, Bolland KJ. (2000, March). A synergistic effect of a daily supplement for 1 month of 200 mg magnesium plus 50 mg vitamin B6 for the relief of anxiety-related premenstrual symptoms: a randomized double-blind crossover study. *J Womens Health Gend Based Med*, (2):131–39.

Durlach J, Pages N, Bac P, Bara M, Guiet-Bara A. (2002, December). Magnesium deficit and sudden infant death syndrome

(SIDS): SIDS due to magnesium deficiency and SIDS due to various forms of magnesium depletion; possible importance of the chronopathological form. *Magnes Res*, 15(3–4):269–78.

Erasmus U. (1986). *Fats and Oils*. Alive Books, Vancouver, Canada.

Ezpeleta L, Keeler G, Erkanli A, Costello EJ, Angold A. (2001, October). Epidemiology of psychiatric disability in childhood and adolescence. *J Child Psychol Psychiatry*, 42(7):901–4.

Fava GA. (2003, February). Can long-term treatment with antidepressant drugs worsen the course of depression? *J Clin Psychiatry*, 64:2 123–33.

Fava M. (2001). Augmentation and combination strategies in treatment-resistant depression. *J Clin Psychiatry*, 62 Suppl 18:4–11.

Fincher CE, Chang TS, Harrel EH, Kettelhut MC, Rea Wj, Johnson A, Hickey DC, Fine SB. (1991, June). Resilience and human adaptability: who rises above adversity? *Am J Occup Ther*, 45(6):493–503.

Foley D, Monjan A, Masaki K, Ross W, Havlik R, White L, Launer L. (2001, December). Daytime sleepiness is associated with 3-year incident dementia and cognitive decline in older Japanese-American men. *J Am Geriat Soc*, 49(12):1628–32.

Fosslien E. (2001, January). Mitochondrial medicine—molecular pathology of defective oxidative phosphorylation. *Ann Clin Lab Sci*, 31(1):25–67.

Fraga Fuentes MD, de Juana Velasco P, Pintor Recusnco R. (1996 July/August). Metabolic role of glutamine and its importance in nutritional therapy. *Nutr Hosp*, 11(4):215–25.

Freeman MP, Freeman SA, McElroy SL. (2002, February). The comorbidity of bipolar and anxiety disorders: prevalence, psychobiology, and treatment issues. *J Affect Disord*, 68(1):1–23.

Fux M, Levine J, Aviv A, Belmaker RH. (1996, September). Inositol treatment of obsessive-compulsive disorder. *Am J Psychiatry*, 153(9)1219–21.

Galland L. (1985). Normocalcemic tetany and candidiasis. *Magnesium*, 4(5–6):339–44.

Ganouni S, Tazi A, Hakkou F. (1998, June). Potential serotonergic interactions with the anxiolytic-like effects of calcium channel antagonists. *Pharmacol Biochem Behav*, 60(2):365–69.

Gehring WJ, Himle J, Nisenson LG. (2001, January). Action-monitoring dysfunction in obsessive-compulsive disorder. *Psychol Sci*, 11(1):1–6.

Gerson MD. (1998). *The Second Brain.* HarperCollins, New York.

Gillin JC, Buchsbaum M, Wu J, Clark C, Bunney W. (2001). Sleep deprivation as a model experimental antidepressant treatment: findings from functional brain imaging. *Depress Anxiety*, 14(1):37–49.

Gobel H, Fresenius J, Heinze A, Dworschak M, Soyka D. (1996, August). Effectiveness of Oleum Menthae Piperitae and Paracetamol in therapy of headache of the tension type. *Nervenarze*, 67(8):672–81.

Gorwood P. (1999, September). From stressful life events to anxiety disorders. *Rev Prat*, 15:49(14)Suppl:S11-3.

Gottfries CG. (2001). Late life depression. *Eur Arch Psychiatry Clin Neurosci*, 251 Suppl 2:1157–61.

Grevet EH, Tietzmann MR, Shansis FM, Hastenpflugl C, Santana LC, Forster L, Kapczinskil F, Izquierdo I. (2002, March). Behavioral effects of acute phenylalanine and tyrosine depletion in healthy male volunteers. *J Psychopharmacol*, 16(1):51–53.

Gupta MB, Nath C, Patuaik GK, Saxena RC. (1996, June). Effect of calcium channel blockers on withdrawal syndrome of lorazepam in rats. *Indian J Med Res*, 103:310–14.

Hall JC, Heel K, McCauley R. (1996 March). Glutamine. *Br J Surg*, 83(3):305–12.

Haller J, Fuchs E, Halasz J, Makara GB. (1999, September). Defeat is a major stressor in males while social instability is stressful mainly in females: towards the development of a social stress model in female rats. *Brain Res Bull*, 1;50(1):33–39.

Hansen CJ, Stevens LC, Coast JR. Exercise duration and mood state: how much is enough to feel better? *Health Psychol*, 2001 (7);20(4):267–75.

Hartman E. (1983). Two case reports: night terrors with sleep-walking—a potentially lethal disorder. *J of Nerv Ment Dis*, 171:37–40.

Hassmen P, Koivula N, Uutela A. Physical exercise and psychological well-being: a population study in Finland. *Preventative Medicine*, 2000(1);30(1):17–25.

Held K, Antonijevic I, Kunzel H, Uhr M, Wetter TC, Golly IC, Steiger A, Murck H. (2002, July). Oral Mg supplementation reverses age-related neuroendocrine and sleep EEG changes in humans. *Pharmacopsychiatry*, 35(4):135–43.

Hettema JM, Annas P, Neale C, Kendler KS, Fredrikson M, Sci M. (2003, July). A Twin Study of the Genetics of Fear Conditioning. *Arch Gen Psych*, 60(7):702–8.

Hirschfield RM. (1996). Panic disorder: diagnosis, epidemiology, and clinical course. *J Clin Psychiatry*, 57 Suppl 10:3–8.

Hollander E, Allen A, Steiner M, Wheadon DE, Oakes R, Burnham DB. (2003, September). Acute and long-term treatment and prevention of relapse of obsessive-compulsive disorder with paroxetine. *J Clin Psychiatry*, 64(9):1113–21.

Ilmberger J, Heuberger E, Mahrhofer C, Dessovic H, Kowarik D, Buchbauer G. (2001, March). The influence of essential oils on human attention, 1: alertness. *Chem Senses*, 26(3):239–45.

Isensee B, Wittchen HU, Stein M, Hofler M, Stat D, Lich R. (2003, July). Smoking increases the risk of panic. *Arch Gen Psychiatry*, 60(7):649–700.

Issberner U, Reeh PW, Steen KH. (1996, April). Pain due to tissue acidosis: a mechanism for inflammatory and ischemic myalgia? *Neurosci Lett*, 26;208(3):191–194.

Jancin B. (2003, February). Think bipolar in treatment-resistant anxiety. *Clin Psych News*, V.31:30.

Jarvis DC. (1958). *Folk Medicine*. Henry Holt, New York.

Jeffery HE, McCleary BV, Hensley WJ, Read DJ. (1985, August). Thiamine deficiency–a neglected problem of infants and mothers–possible relationship to sudden infant death syndrome. *Aust NZ Obstet Gynaecol*, 25(3):198–202.

Johns MW, Dudley HA, Masterton JP. (1976, May). The sleep habits, personality and academic performance of medical students. *Med. Educ*, 10(3):158–62.

Juntunen J, Teravainen H, Eriksson K, Larsen A, Hillbom M. (1979, August). Peripheral neuropathy and myopathy. An experimental study of rats on alcohol and variable dietary thiamine. *Virchows Arch A Pathol Anat Histol*, 23;383(3):241–52.

Kail M. (2002, August). The relationship between physical activity, health status and psychological well-being of fertility-aged women. *Scan J Med Sci Sports*, 12(4):241–47.

Kane M. (2002). *The Botox Book*. St. Martin's Press, New York.

Kapar VK (2002, May). The relationship between chronically disrupted sleep and healthcare use. *Sleep*, 1;25(3):289–96.

Karol MH, Macina OT, Cunningham A. (2001, December). Cell and molecular biology of chemical allergy. *Ann Allergy Asthma Immunol*, 87(6 Suppl 3):28–32.

Kipen HM, Fiedler N. (2000, April). A 37-year-old mechanic with multiple chemical sensitivities. *Environ Health Perspect*, 108(4):377–81.

Koopman C, Classen C, Cardena E, Spiegel D. (1995, January). When disaster strikes, acute stress disorder may follow. *J Trauma Stress*, 8(1):29–46.

Kowald A. (2001, May/August). The mitochondrial theory of aging. *Biol Signals Recept*. 10(3–4):162–75.

Kozlovskii VL, Mosin AE, Ivakina LV. (1996, January). The effect of the subchronic administration of calcium-channel blockers on CNS excitability. *Eksp Klin Farmakol*, 59(1):14–16.

Krahn LE. (2003, August). A new way to treat narcolepsy. *Current Psychiatry*, 2(8):65–69.

Kuloglu M, Atmaca M, Tezcan E, Gecici O, Tunckol H, Ustundag H. (2002). Antioxidant enzyme activities and malondialdehyde levels with patients with obsessive-compulsive disorder. *Neuropsychobiology*, 46(1):27–32.

Kurt TL. (1995). Multiple chemical sensitivities–a syndrome of pseudotoxicity manifest as exposure perceived symptoms. *J Toxicol Clin Toxicol*, 33(2):101–5.

Langohr HD, Petruch F, Schroth G. (1981). "Vitamin B_1, B_2 and B_6 deficiency in neurological disorders. *J. Neurol*, 225(2):95–108.

Lempereur L, Cantarella G, Marabito P, Chiarenza A, Fiore L, Sappala G, Bernardini R. (1999, October). Thymic hormones, cancer and behavioral adaptive responses. *Ann Med*, 31 Suppl 2:40–45.

Lepine JP. (2002). The epidemiology of anxiety disorders: prevalence and societal costs. *J Clin Psychiatry*, 63 Suppl 14:4–8.

Lichodziejewska B, Klos J, Rezler J, Grudzka K, Dluzniewska M, Rudaj A, Ceremuzynski L. (2002, September). Clinical symptoms of mitral valve prolapse are related to hypomagnesemia and attenuated by magnesium. *Biophys Chem*, 99(1):63.

Lindberg E, Carter N, Janson C. (2001, December). Role of snoring and daytime sleepiness in occupational accidents. *Am J Respir Crit Care Med*, 1;164(11):2031–35.

Lonsdale D. (1990). Asymmetric functional dysautonomia. *J Nutr Med*, 1:254–64.

Lonsdale D. (1990, February). Hypothesis and case reports: possible thiamine deficiency. *J Am Coll Nutr*, 9(1):13–17.

Lonsdale D, Shamberger RJ. (1980). Red cell transketolase as an indicator of nutritional deficiency. *Am J Clin Nut*, 33:205–11.

Macias-Matos C, Rodriquez-Ojea A, Chi N, Jimenez S, Zulueta D, Bates CJ. (1996, September). "Biochemical evidence of thiamine depletion during the Cuban neuropathy epidemic, 1992–1993." *Am. J. Clin. Nutr*, 64(3):347–53.

Mahoney DJ, Parise G, Tarnopolsky MA. (2002, November).

Nutritional and exercise-based therapies in the treatment of mitochondrial disease. *Curr Opin Clin Nutr Metab Care*, 5(6):619–29.

Mallon L, Broman JE, Hetta K. (2002, March). Sleep complaints predict coronary artery disease mortality in males: a 12 year follow-up study of a middle-age, Swedish population. *Intern Med*, 251(3):207–16.

McConachie I, Haskew A. (1998). "Thiamine status after major trauma." *Intensive Care Med*, 14(6):628–31.

Mehta KM, Simonsick EM, Penninx WH, Schultz R, Rubin SM, Satterfield S, Yaffe K. (2003, April). Prevalence and correlates of anxiety symptoms in well functioning older adults: findings from the Health Aging and Body Composition Study. *J Am Geriat Soc*, 51(4):449.

Melchior CL, Ritzmann RF. (1994, March). Dehydroepiandrosterone is an anxiolytic in mice on the plus maze. *Pharmacol Biochem Behav*, 47(3):437–41.

Moritz S, Birkner C, Kloss M, Jahn H, Hand I, Haasen C, Krausz. (2002, July). Executive functioning in obsessive-compulsive disorder, unipolar depression and schizophrenia. *Arch Clin Neuropsychol*, 17(5):477–83.

Mosqueria M, Iturriage R. (2002, August). Carotid body chemosensory excitation induced by nitric oxide: involvement of oxidative metabolism. *Respir Physiol Neurobiol*, 1;131(3):175–87.

Moss R, D'Amico S, Maletta G. (1987, December). Mental dysfunction as a sign of organic illness in the elderly. *Geriatrics*, 42(12): 35–42.

Nahas Z. (March, 2003). Vagus nerve stimulation the next breakthrough for treatment of resistant depression? *Psychiatric Times*.

Nascimento I, Nardi AE, Valenca AM, Lopes FL, Mezzalma MA, Nascentes, R, Zin WA. (2002, May). Psychiatric disorders in asthmatic outpatients. *Psychiatry Res*, 15;110(1):73–80.

Nava F, Carta G. (2001, July). Melatonin reduces anxiety induced by lipopolysaccharide in the rat. *Neurosci Lett*, 6;307(1):57–60.

Neziruglu F, McKay D, Yuryura-Tobias JA. (2000, November/

December). Overlapping and distinctive features of hypochondriasis and obsessive-compulsive disorder. *J Anxiety Disord*, 14(6):603–14.

Obut TA, Lipina TV, Koriakina LA, Kudriavtseva NN. (2001, July/August). Is dehydroepiandrosterone sulfate an anxiolytic agent? *Zh Vyssh Nerv Deiat Im I P Pavlova*, 51(4):502–6.

Okun MS, McDonald WM, DeLong MR. (2002, May). Refractory nonmotor symptoms in male patients with Parkinson disease due to testosterone deficiency: a common unrecognized comorbidity. *Arch Neurol*, 59(5):807–11.

Ostrovskii AA, Nikitin VS. (1985, July/August). Posttraumatic regeneration of the skeletal muscles in certain forms of hypovitaminosis B_1. *Vopr Pitan*, (4):48–51.

Paladiai AC. (1995, June) Apigenin, a component of Matricari recutita flowers, is a central benzodiazepine receptor-ligand with anxiolytic effects. *Planta Med*, 61(3):213–16.

Paladiai AC, Marder M, Viola H, Wolfman C, Wasowski C, Medina JH. (1999, May). Flavonoids and the central nervous system: from forgotten factors to potent anxiolytic compounds. *J Pharm Pharmaco*, 51(5):519–26.

Palataik A, Frolov K, Fux M, Benjamin J. (2001, June). Double-blind, controlled, crossover trial of inositol versus fluvoxamine for the treatment of panic disorder. *J Clin Psychopharmacol*. 21(3):335–39.

Papp LA, et al. (1997, November). Respiratory psychophysicology of panic disorder: three respiratory challenges in 98 subjects. *Am J Psychiatry*, 154(11):1557–65.

Peters RA, Thompson RH. (1975, June). Pyruvic acid as an intermediary metabolite in the brain tissue of avitaminous and normal pigeons. *Nutr Rev*, 33(7):211–12.

Philbert R, Caspers K, Langbehn D, Troughton EP, Yucuis R, Sandhu HK, Cadoret RJ. (2002, September/October). The association of a HOPA polymorphism with major depression and phobia. *Compr Psychiatry*, 43(5):404–10.

Prasad A, Prasad C. (1996, September). Short-term consumption of a diet rich in fat decreases anxiety response in adult male rats. *Physiol Behav*, 60(3):1039–42.

Ray US, Mukhopadhyaya S, Purkayastha SS, Asnani V, Tomer OS, Prashad R, et al. Effect of yogic exercises on physical and mental health of young fellowship course trainees. *Ind J Physio Pharm*, 2001(1);45(1):37–53.

Regier DA, Narrow WE, Rae DS. (1990). The epidemiology of anxiety disorders: the Epidemiologic Catchment Area (ECA) experience. *J Psychiatr Res*, 24 Suppl 2:3–14.

Riolo S. Poster session American Academy of Child and Adolescent Psychiatry. 49th annual meeting, October 2002.

Ross GH, Rea WJ, Johnson AR, Hickey DC, Simon TR. (1999, April/June). Neurotoxicity in single photon emission computed tomography brain scans of patients reporting chemical sensitivities. *Toxicol Ind Health*, 15(3–4):415–20.

Roth T. (2001, January). The relationship between psychiatric disease and insomnia. *Int J Clin Pract Suppl*, 116:3–8.

Rouch PK, Stern D. (1986, January). Life threatening injuries resulting from sleepwalking and night terrors. *Psychosomatics*, 27:62–64.

Rupprecht R, Holsboer F. (2001). Neuroactive steroids in neuropsychopharmacology. *Int Rev Neurobiol*, 46:461–77.

Rupprecht R, Michele F, Hermann B, Strohle A, Lancel M, Romero E, Hobboer F. (2001, November). Neuroactive steroids: molecular mechanisms of action and implications for neuropsychopharmacology. *Brain Res Rev*, 37(1–3):59–67.

Sagduyu K. (2003, March). Omega 3 fatty acids. *Psychiatric Times*.

Sarkisova KYu, Kulikov MA. (2001, September/October). Prophylactic actions of the antioxidant agent AEKOL on behavioral disturbances induced by chronic stress in rats. *Neurosci Behav Physiol*, 31(5):503–8.

Schwartau M, Doehn M. (1981, September). Metabolic acidosis caused by thiamin deficiency. *Anaesthesist*, 30(9):452–54.

Seelig MS. (1994, October). Consequences of magnesium deficiency on the enhancement of stress reactions; preventive and therapeutic implications. *J Am Coll Nutr*, 13(5):429–46.

Simon NM, Blacker D, Korbly NB, Sharma SG, Worthington JJ, Otto MW, Pollack MH. (2002, May). Hypothyroidism and hyperthyroidism in anxiety disorders revisited: new data and literature review. *J Affect Disord*, 69(1–3):209–17.

Simon TR. (1997, January). Comparison of single photon emission computed tomography finding in cases of healthy adults and solvent-exposed adults. *Am J Ind Med*, 31(1):4–14.

Simon TR, Hickey DC, Fincher CE, Johnson AR, Ross GH, Rea WJ. (1990, August). Single photon emission computed tomography of the brain in patients with chemical sensitivities. *Pharmacol Biochem Behav*, 36(4):997–1000.

Sinoff G, Werner P. (2003). "Anxiety, Depression and Cognitive Impairment: What Precedes What in This Intricate Triad?" 2003 lecture at the University of Haifa, Israel. Smith JC, O'Connor PJ, Crabbe JB, Dishman RK. (2002, July). Emotional responsiveness after low and moderate-intensity exercise and seated rest. *Med Sci Sports Exerc*, 34(7):1158–67.

Smriga M, Torii K. (2003, April). Prolonged treatment with L-lysine and L-arginine reduces stress induced anxiety in an elevated plus maze. *Nutrit Neurosci*, 6(2):125–28.

Sogduyuk. (2002, November/December). Peppermint oil for irritable bowel syndrome. *Psychosomatics*, 43(6):508–9.

Souba WW, Klimberg VS, Plumley DA, Salloum RM, Flynn TC, Bland KI, Copeland EM. (1990, April). The role of glutamine in maintaining a healthy gut and supporting the metabolic response to injury and infection. *J Surg Res*, 48(4):383–91.

Steen KH, Steen AE, Kreysel HW, Reeh PW. (1996, August). "Inflammatory mediators potentiate pain induced by experimental tissue acidosis." *Pain*, 66(2–3):163–70.

Tarlo SM, Poonai N, Binkley K, Antony MM, Swinson RP. (2002, August). Responses to panic induction procedures in subjects with multiple chemical sensitivity/idiopathic environmental intolerance; understanding the relationship with panic disorder. *Environ Health Perspect*, 110 Suppl 4:669–71.

Tate S. (1997, September). Peppermint oil: a treatment for postoperative nausea. *J Adv Nurs*, 26(3):343–49.

Tate T, Petruzzello K. (1995, December). Negative feelings are decreased by aerobic exercises while positive feelings are significantly increased. *J Sports Med Phys Fitness*, 35(4):295–302.

Tietzel AJ, Lack LC. (2001, May). The short term benefits of brief and long naps following nocturnal sleep restriction. *Sleep*, 1;24(3):293–300.

Towbin KE, Lockman JF, Cohen DJ. (1987, Spring). Drug treatment of obsessive-compulsive disorders: a review of findings in the light of diagnostic and metric limitations. *Psychiatr Dev*, 5(1):25–50.

Umezu T, Sakata A, Ito H. (2001, July/August). Ambulation-promoting effect of peppermint oil and identification of its active constituents. *Pharmacol Biochem Behav*, 69(3–4):383–90.

Verburg K, Griez E, Meijer J, Pols H. (2002, July). Discrimination between panic disorder and generalized anxiety disorder by 35% carbon dioxide challenge. *Am J Psychiatry*, 1;152(7):1081–83.

Walker AF, De Souza MC, Vickers MF, Abeyasekera S, Collins ML, Trinca LA. (1998, November). Magnesium supplementation alleviates premenstrual symptoms of fluid retention. *J Women's Health*, (9):157–65.

Wei YH, Lu CY, Lee GD, Pang CY, Ma YS. (1998, November). Oxidative damage and mutation to mitochondrial DNA and age-dependent decline of mitochondrial respiratory function. *Ann N Y Acad Sci*, 20;854:155–70.

Weisskopf MG, Chen H, Schwarzschild MA, Kawachi I, Ascherio A. (2003, June). Prospective study of phobic anxiety and risk of Parkinson's disease. *Mov Disord*, 18(6):646–51.

Whitehus MJ, Li N, Zhang M, Wang M, Horwitz MA, Nelson SK, Horwitz LD, Brechun N. (2002, March). Thiol antioxidants inhibit the adjuvant effects of aerosolized diesel exhaust particles in a murine model for ovalbumin sensitization. *J Immunol*, 1;168(5): 2560.

Wittchen HU, Krause P, Hofler M. Pittrow D. Winter S, Spiegel B, Hajak G, Riemann D, Steiger A, Pfister H. (2001). The "Nationwide Insomnia Screening and Awareness Study." Prevalence and interventions in primary care. *Fortschr Med Orig*, 119(1):9–19.

Wolfman C, Viola H, Paladini A, Dajas F, Medina JH. (1994, January). Possible anxiolytic effects of chrysin, a central benzodiazepine receptor ligand isolated from Passiflora coerulea. *Pharmacol Biochem Behav*, 47(1):1–4.

Xu F, Zhang Y, Lou Y. (1998, August). Effects of different thyroid status on the pharmacokinetics of diazepam. *Yao Xue Xue Bao*, 33(8):571–75.

Zamm AV. (1995, January). Successful treatment of universal reactors with prophylactic aspirin—a preliminary report. *J Ortho Med*, 3;88:44–46.

Zito JM. (2003, January). *Arch Pediatr Adolesc Med*, 157(1):17–25.

Index